YOGA FOR FLEXIBILITY, STRENGTH AND BALANCE

A Practical Structured Guide

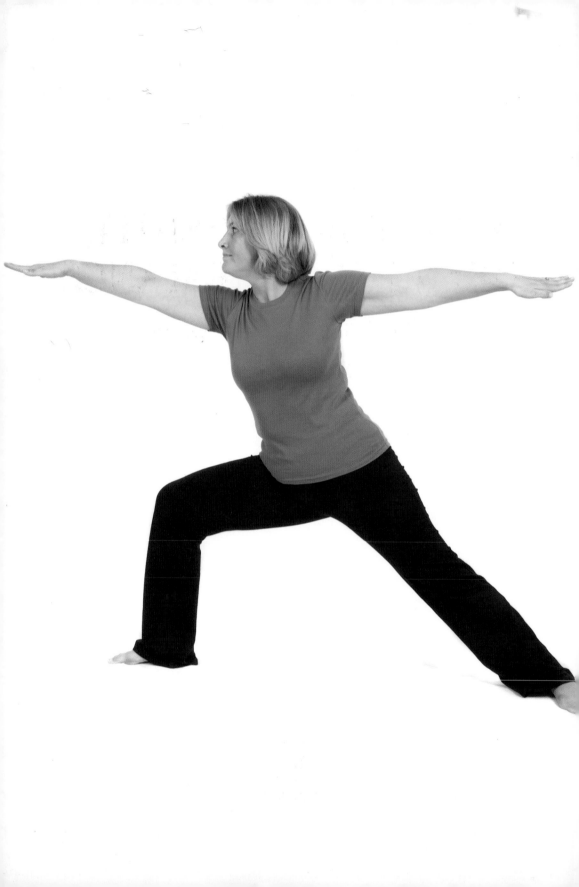

YOGA FOR FLEXIBILITY, STRENGTH AND BALANCE

A Practical Structured Guide

Nita A. Martin

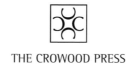

THE CROWOOD PRESS

First published in 2009 by
The Crowood Press Ltd
Ramsbury, Marlborough
Wiltshire SN8 2HR

www.crowood.com

British Library Cataloguing-in-Publication Data
A catalogue record for this book is available from the British Library.

ISBN 978 1 84797 080 0

Disclaimer
Whilst every effort has been made to ensure that the content of this book is as
technically accurate as possible, neither the author nor the publishers can
accept responsibility for any injury or loss sustained as a result of the use of
this material. It is the responsibility of the individual to ensure that they are fit
to participate and they should seek medical advice from a qualified
professional where appropriate.

Acknowledgements
Thanks to Andrew Kuc and Karen Cox for taking part in the photo shoot and
to Kevin Wood for the photography.

Designed and typeset by Focus Publishing,
11a St Botolph's Road, Sevenoaks, Kent TN

Printed and bound in Malaysia by Times Offset (M) Sdn Bhd

Contents

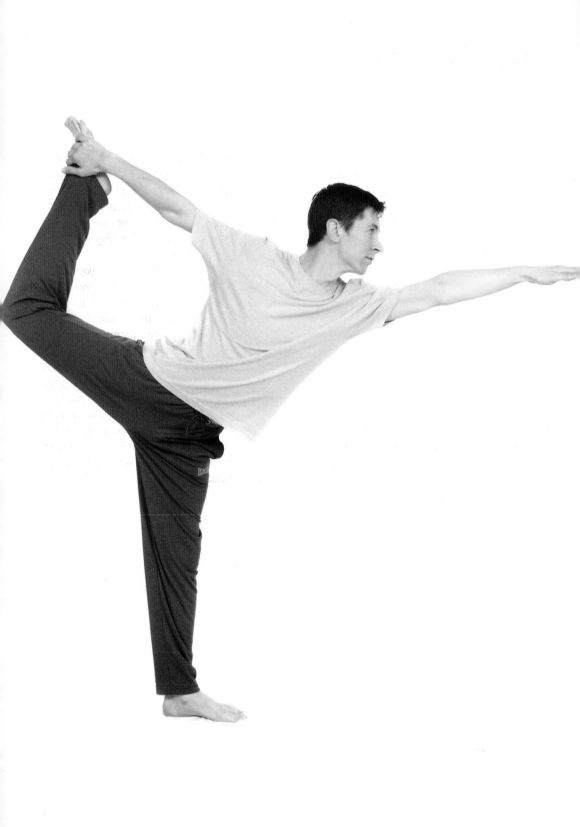

Introduction

Fitness is not just defined by how far or how fast you can run or by how much weight you can lift. Flexibility is also an integral part of being fit. Training in yoga is an excellent way to work towards improving your flexibility. Not only that, but yoga will also help you to develop your strength and balance. To maintain your range of movement, your body needs to be regularly taken through its full range. If this does not happen, then a loss of flexibility can occur and, in some cases, this can be permanent. So, for the best results, you should incorporate a regular training programme into your life sooner rather than later. Saying that, it is never too late to get started and any training that you do will benefit you.

Simple stretching exercises have long been a mandatory part of training programmes for athletes. An increasing level of importance, however, is being placed on stretching as a way of maintaining a healthy body and mind, reducing muscle fatigue and injury and improving overall performance. Due to this change in emphasis, a number of exercises from yoga have increasingly been incorporated into normal sports training, often without the participants realizing that what they are doing are actually yoga poses.

This book brings together classic yoga exercises and stretching training and presents a structured programme that can be used for improving individual understanding and development. Together they form an essential guide to stretching: Yoga for flexibility, strength and balance. It is a useful companion both to newcomers to yoga training and also to more advanced students who are looking for more challenging poses to perform. This chapter introduces the structured approach and gives a short description of the material covered within each chapter and how it can be used.

A Structured Approach

The approach taken in this book is focused on developing flexibility, strength and balance through a structured programme. Simple, step by step instructions are given for each exercise and pose. These intermediate steps form perfect exercises for developing the body in order to achieve the full pose. The steps are shown in order of increasing difficulty and so they can be used to establish your ability level and range of motion with respect to each individual exercise.

Being able to complete one pose successfully, you may be surprised to find that you cannot complete a similar looking pose. It is not always possible to predict how you will fare with an exercise without giving it a go. In this way, yoga training is very much a personal journey. Looking at it another way, these steps also show you how to adapt the exercises to match your ability level and range of motion. Not only that, but working your way through each step until you reach the one that represents your level will act as a brilliant way to prepare the muscles that are required for each pose. Therefore, it is recommended that during training you should take your time and work through each step successively rather than going straight to the step that represents the maximum that you can achieve.

These step by step instructions can also be used to track your progress. By making a note of the date that you can achieve each progressive step, these steps can be used to motivate you in your training, since you will be able to identify your progress clearly as well as seeing what you will eventually be able to achieve with continued training.

Yoga practice requires much patience and perseverance as improvements in ability can be slow and gradual. It is hoped that this book will encourage you to work towards mastering the poses and exercises shown.

Using the Step by Step Instructions

The step by step pictures and instructions presented in this book can be used in a number of ways to:

- Establish your range of motion
- Establish your ability to balance and hold positions requiring strength
- Prepare to perform the complete pose
- Motivate you by showing you what comes next
- Track progress

Flexibility

Fitness training is not just about how fast you can run or how much weight you can lift. There are many components to fitness and flexibility is just one of them. Your flexibility is your ability to bend – your range of movement around a joint. Flexibility can be both maintained and improved through stretching and yoga can help you to achieve just that.

If the body is not regularly taken through its full range of movement, then a loss in flexibility will be experienced. Additionally, imbalances in the body may be introduced through a lack of specific training that together can increase the risk of muscle injury and muscle pain, such as back pain. Without regular training, the muscles can shorten and permanent loss of flexibility can occur. The earlier in life one starts training, the more these negative effects can be delayed or indeed reversed, as everyday movements alone will probably not be sufficient to take your body through the training it needs to remain fully supple.

Breaks in yoga training quickly result in a loss of flexibility. The training presented in this book is an excellent way in which to incorporate regular stretching into your life. In addition, such training can be used to enhance sporting performance for athletes through the identification of which muscles and movements are needed for a particular sport and working on the poses that develop them. This can help to reduce the risk of injury. For this reason, yoga training is an excellent activity for complementing all forms of sports training. Most importantly, improving your flexibility will help you to feel younger for longer.

There is a large variation in ability when it comes to flexibility, as you will be able to see whenever you attend a yoga class. Each individual has a specific history and so each individual has specific levels of flexibility. Simple things like how you sit each day, what activities and sports you do and any injuries that you have had in the past can all influence your flexibility and so no two individuals will be alike. It is not uncommon to find that students are unable to do simple exercises that they could do when they were younger, such as kneeling or turning their head to look behind them. This should not be a discouragement in any way from training, but rather a stage of self-awareness to help create a more suitable training programme that fits your needs.

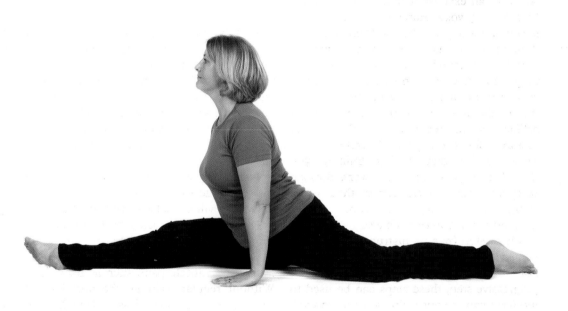

Yoga pose requiring flexibility: the Hanuman (monkey god) pose.

Strength

Strength is a component of fitness that is not immediately associated with yoga. And yet, when it comes to practising yoga, lack of strength can easily be the sole reason for not being able to master a pose. It is not enough to be able to get into a pose momentarily, you must be able to hold and feel comfortable in the pose in order to have truly mastered it. Poses such as the plank pose require much body weight to be supported on the arms and hence arm strength is required. Strength is needed to enable you to hold many of the exercises presented in this book. For this reason, they can help you to develop your strength by training towards holding these poses for increasing amounts of time.

Holding positions that require balance is tiring work and this is where strength often comes into play. The stronger your muscles, the longer you will be able to maintain the balancing pose. It is not unusual for these poses to work the muscles the hardest and students often find themselves sweating and out of breath after such a workout.

Balance

Balance is another component of fitness that is not immediately associated with yoga. And yet, when it comes to practising yoga, a lack of balance can also easily be the sole reason for not being able to master a pose. Poses such as the double toe hold pose

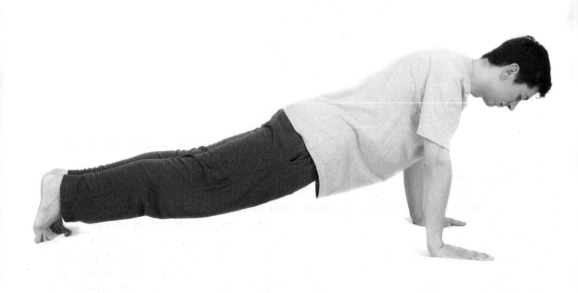

Yoga pose requiring strength: the plank pose.

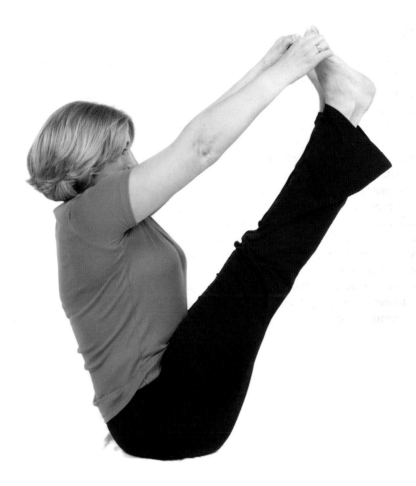

Yoga pose requiring balance: the double toe hold pose.

are difficult because they require you to balance on your bottom. When you first attempt this pose, you may well find that you keel over backwards. It will take some practice in order to be able to hold this pose for some time without falling over. Balance is required to enable you to hold many of the exercises presented in this book. Therefore, they can also help you to develop your balance by training towards holding these poses for increasing amounts of time. Balancing poses in this book come in a variety of forms, ranging from balancing on one leg to balancing on one leg and one arm. They can be very satisfying to perform once mastered.

Balancing will require you to have a sense of your centre of gravity and will also need you to continually adjust the usage of your muscles and your alignment in order to hold the pose. Simple techniques can be used to help you, such as focusing your gaze on a steady point, slightly bending at the knees, widening your base or even starting by supporting yourself against a wall. The latter may help you to achieve the pose fully while using the wall to help you balance. All of these things will give you greater stability.

How to Use this Book

Chapter 1: History of Yoga

This chapter looks at the origins of yoga going back over 4,000 years and up to the present day. The earliest references to yoga are found in ancient Hindu scriptures. This chapter looks briefly at the pathway of yoga to current day practice as it has been documented through these scriptures. Yoga practice is not just about performing postures. This is just how it has become known and popularized in the West. Achieving a steady mind and preparing the individual for spiritual enlightenment were the original aims and there are a number of yoga pathways that can be taken to achieve this goal. The practice of postures is just one of them.

It is not necessary for students to know about the origins of yoga right from the start in order to enjoy the training. However, such knowledge can help students to choose the right 'type' of yoga for them and may help to increase their enjoyment. Whereas some yoga poses, for example, are literally named, describing the exercise performed precisely, others are named through dedications to gods or to heroes and so a little knowledge about the background of yoga practice will help you to appreciate these characteristics.

Chapter 2: Guide for Beginners

It is not unusual for students to be nervous about getting started with training. Often they worry about whether they are flexible enough to join a class. There is no minimum level for getting started. Regular practice is what will make your training successful. Yoga is not a competitive sport. So, do not judge yourself against others. Only focus on what you can do and how you can develop. Give yourself the time that your body needs.

This chapter presents recommendations on how best to train and also gives some training tips. The poses in this book are presented in a step by step way. This is so that you can find the appropriate step that you can achieve and work on before moving onto progressively harder steps and eventually mastering the complete pose. This chapter discusses how you can use this book to:

• Establish your range of motion
• Plan sessions to meet your development needs
• Modify exercises to suit your ability level
• Track your progress

It is important to train safely and not to train through pain and injury. Common contraindications to training are presented in this chapter. It is always best to seek professional medical advice if you have any concerns.

Yoga does not require much in terms of equipment. Loose clothing will make practice more comfortable and a training mat will help you to define your training space and provide support for more difficult poses. Other types of training equipment that are available include blocks and straps, and this chapter discusses when it may be appropriate to consider these various aids.

Chapter 3: Your Body and Yoga

Although training in yoga does not require a detailed understanding of how the muscles and joints work, it can certainly be useful to have some basic knowledge as this will increase your appreciation of your training. Many students often ask about what exercises will help certain muscles and also which muscles are being worked in any given exercise. This chapter will help the student to identify the parts of the body that they are developing through their training and in any particular exercise. In addition, knowing where the muscles are, how they connect to the bones and how each of the major joints work can give you a better indication of the potential to be gained from each exercise.

Yoga instructors will tend to check your alignment and posture and this is to do with ensuring that you are working the correct muscles for that particular exercise and performing exercises in a way that will reduce the risk of injury. If, for example, your leg is slightly rotated rather than being straight, then you will be working the leg muscles in a different way to what the pose intended. Sometimes incorrect alignment over many repetitions of an exercise may cause discomfort and even eventually lead to an increased risk of injury.

This chapter presents a basic introduction to both skeletal and muscular structure in relation to stretching and contracting the muscles during yoga exercises. It describes the different stages of muscle contraction and also how to describe movement. There are a number of different ways to stretch: static, active, PNF (proprioceptive neuro-muscular facilitation) and ballistic stretching. (The safest methods of training are considered to be a combination of static and PNF stretching.) These are described in this chapter and you should be aware of what type of stretching you are doing when you are training.

The following detailed illustrations are included in this chapter, to be used as easy reference guides to complement your training.

• The skeletal and muscular systems
• Different types of joints and defining movement
• Types of stretching

Chapters 4–8: The Exercise Chapters

The exercise chapters form the bulk of the material in this book. Each chapter is named according to the type of training included and presents a selection of exercises:

4   Preparation Exercises
5   Seated Exercises
6   Standing Exercises
7   Supine Exercises
8   Floor Exercises

Each exercise is shown using pictures and instructions of each of the steps required to get into a pose, accompanied by a short description of which muscles the pose works and also, where appropriate, teaching points and safety tips. These chapters together form the fully illustrated stretching programme. Variations of poses are also shown that can make the pose either easier or more difficult.

Chapter 9: Session Planning

This chapter will help you start putting together a session that meets your individual development requirements. Having used the exercises in the previous chapters to evaluate your ability level and development needs, you can then use the session planner to create sessions appropriate to you. This is a great way to get started in forming your own training plan and it can be adjusted to meet your needs as time goes on.

The session planner is designed by considering each session to consist of four stages: preparation, fundamentals, challenge and relaxation. How long you spend on each stage and what exercises each stage comprises is down to you. A number of stage samples are presented in the session planner, providing quick reference guides for use during your own planning and training.

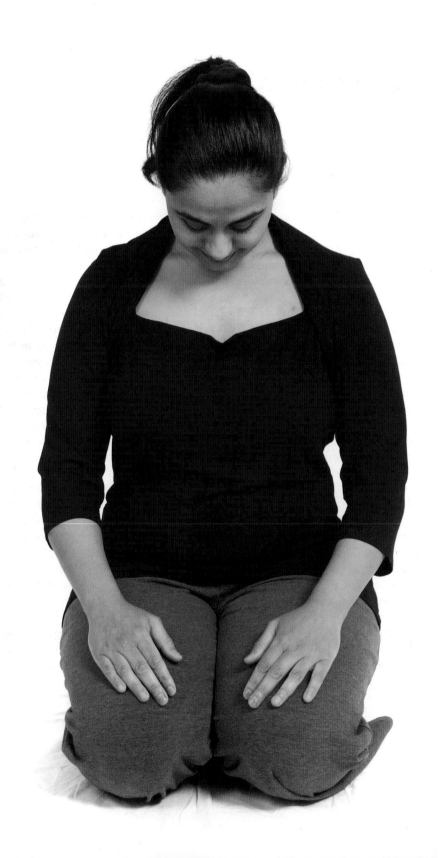

1   History of Yoga

Yoga is a very old practice that originally used physical exercises and meditation to prepare the individual for seeking spiritual enlightenment. Today, yoga in the West is predominantly concerned with postures and breathing exercises as a way of improving physical and emotional health. It has mostly been removed from its original spiritual practice and aims. Back in India, however, where yoga originated, the practice of yoga as a search for spiritual enlightenment remains commonplace, particularly among Hindu priests.

The origins of this practice may be of great interest to you as a beginner; or the opposite may be true and your foremost interest lies in starting to reap the benefits of improving your physical well-being. Whichever the case, however, it can be useful to know the context from which yoga originated as it may aid you in selecting the right 'type' of yoga for you and increase your enjoyment of it.

Yoga has many meanings, changing over time as well as with context, which can make it difficult to comprehend. Here we define yoga as a method of steadying the mind and look into its roots, which are steeped deep in Indian history and tradition. Yoga is not just about physical exercise: this is just one of the many forms that yoga practice can take.

The earliest references to yoga have been found in the excavations in the Indus Valley and are considered to be more than 4,000 years old. These are in the form of pictures and seals of individuals in commonly recognized yoga positions, such as the lotus pose. The earliest written references are found in ancient Hindu scriptures going as far back as 3,500 years. The Vedas, for example, describe the practice of yoga as a pathway to steadying the mind. The Bhagavad Gita (c. 500 BC) is considered to be the most important scripture discussing yoga philosophy. However, it is Patanjali's Yoga Sutras (200 BC) that are attributed with presenting a systemized and standardized form of yoga. Patanjali founded the eight stages of yoga, also know as Ashtanga yoga. This form of yoga is considered to focus on the spiritual aspect of yoga, separating it from the physical aspect. It was only much later that the importance of physical training was rekindled: the Hatha Yoga Pradipika, for example, composed in the fifteenth century, focused on physical training in order to prepare the body for spiritual training and eventual spiritual enlightenment.

Yoga's modern day popularity in the West is largely due to the yoga instructors who travelled to the US and Europe from India in the twentieth century. The Hatha yoga form has become the most popular in the West today and much training focuses on the practice of yoga poses.

Yoga for Steadying the Mind

Yoga is a word from Sanskrit, the ancient Indo-European literary language of India. It has many meanings, but it is commonly interpreted as 'joining' or 'uniting'. A more useful definition is that of it being a pathway for achieving a steady mind. A stillness of the mind can be experienced through the practice of yoga postures and this state can become easier to achieve with training. When focusing on a particular position, the mind leaves all other thoughts and focuses on the moment. Even though these other thoughts and worries may eventually return, training enables you to be released from them at least for a while.

In the West, yoga is commonly associated with the practice of physical poses, and such practice is indeed one of the pathways to achieving a steady mind. The term yoga does not, however, refer to the achievement of this state exclusively through physical exercise. There are a number of other pathways that have been described through various ancient Hindu scriptures and it is through these that the history and development of yoga can be followed. The Vedas, the Upanishads, the Bhagavad Gita, Patanjali's Yoga Sutras and the Hatha Yoga Pradipika all feature within the history of yoga.

Indus Valley Civilization (2000–1000 BC)

If you have had the opportunity to study the early civilizations in world history, then you may well have come across the sites at Mohenjo-daro and Harappa and the Indus Valley civilization, which would have covered most of present day Pakistan and the Western States of India all the way down to Gujarat.

Here archaeological excavations have uncovered the earliest material references to yoga. Most commonly these artefacts are pictures and seals depicting humans or gods meditating in what could be identified as a yoga pose, including the elegant lotus sitting position. Through these discoveries, yoga has been dated as being at least 4,000 years old. It is possible, however, that yoga itself is actually older still. Further detailed information can be found in Vivian Worthington's *A History of Yoga* (1982), which ranges from its beginnings through to the 1900s.

The Vedas (1500–500 BC) and the Upanishads (800–400 BC)

Although yoga is believed to be more than 4,000 years old, the earliest written references to yoga are found in the Vedas, the oldest sacred scriptures of Hinduism, which have been dated as being 3,500 to 2,500 years old. Veda is commonly translated from Sanskrit as 'knowledge'. The Vedas are a collection of poems written in Sanskrit that encompass a system of Hindu philosophy.

The Vedic period is defined as the period in India's history when the Vedas were being composed. These Vedas took the form of teachings and the yoga of this time was known as Vedic yoga. The emphasis of Vedic yoga was on reaching the highest level of spiritual enlightenment through rituals, sacrifices and ceremonies. Vedic yogis, the practitioners of this type of yoga, were responsible for disseminating these teachings. They believed that divine harmony could be reached through self-sacrifice and intense spiritual practice, and it was for this reason that Vedic yogis lived in seclusion in the jungles of India.

A selection from the Vedas called the Upanishads, consisting of 200 scriptures, is considered to mark the end of the Vedic period. They are thought to have been

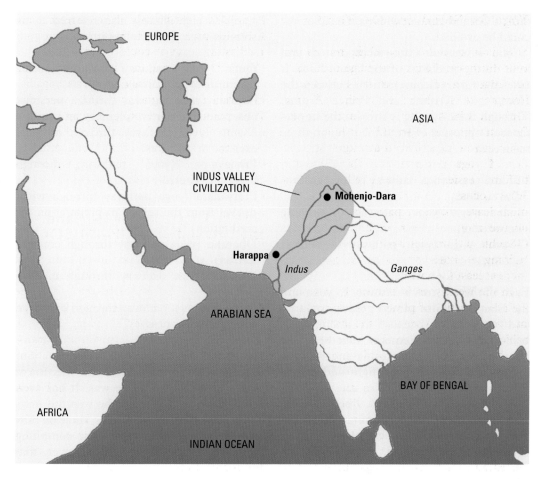

The earliest known references to yoga have been found at the sites of Mohenjo-daro and Harappa in the Indus Valley and are considered to be at least 4,000 years old.

compiled between about 800 BC and 400 BC, although some parts may have been written even later than that. Learnings from the Vedas on meditation and other yoga practices are discussed in the Upanishads, focusing on three key areas:

- Brahman (the universal spirit)
- Atman (the individual soul)
- The relationship between Brahman and Atman

The Bhagavad Gita (500 BC)

The oldest known scripture devoted entirely to yoga is the Bhagavad Gita (its title meaning 'the Lord's song'). It was created around 2,500 years ago and is considered the most important authority on yoga philosophy. It is a part of the Mahabharata, one of the great epics of ancient India. The main teaching of the Bhagavad Gita was that the purpose of being alive was to be active and selfless, and through this way of living,

17

difficulties and contact with pain and sorrow could be avoided.

The Bhagavad Gita incorporated and built on the teachings of the Upanishads. It takes the form of conversations between the Hindu god Krishna and Prince Arjuna. Through these stories, it stresses the importance of opposing evil and focusing on three main areas:

• Bhakti yoga (yoga pathway of loving devotion to God)
• Jnana yoga (yoga pathway of seeking knowledge)
• Karma yoga (yoga pathway of selfless actions)

Each of these forms a pathway to yoga and the Bhagavad Gita gained great popularity and importance because it attempts to bring these three elements together. The conversations between Arjuna and Krishna focus on how Arjuna can fight and escape the bonds that tie him to the material world, the aim being to liberate both himself and his soul. Krishna explains that it is through the yogic training of these three elements that spiritual freedom can be achieved.

Patanjali's Yoga Sutras (200 BC)

Around 200 BC Patanjali attempted to systemize and standardize yoga. He created an eight-limbed (or staged) system of yoga that provided much structure around the practice. He described these stages in his written work, the Yoga Sutras, translated from Sanskrit as the 'threads of yoga', where a sutra is the term meaning an aphoristic rule on rituals and philosophy.

These eight limbs or pathways were individual routes that could be taken to achieve Raja yoga, or control over the mind.

Patanjali's eight limbs, also referred to as Ashtanga yoga, are as follows:

• Yama (yoga pathway through social restraints or ethical values)
• Niyama (yoga pathway through personal observance of purity, tolerance and study)
• Asanas (yoga pathway through physical exercise or postures)
• Pranayama (yoga pathway through breathing control)
• Pratyahara (yoga pathway through withdrawal from the senses in preparation for meditation)
• Dharana (yoga pathway through concentration)
• Dhyana (yoga pathway through meditation)
• Samadhi (yoga pathway through a state of superconsciousness)

Very little is known for certain about Patanjali: where and when he was born, how he lived and who he was. It has even been questioned whether he was the original author of the Yoga Sutras, since he may have only been responsible for compiling them. It cannot be denied, however, that the Yoga Sutras formed the basis of much modern yoga. Previous scriptures had believed that matter and spirit needed to be unified to achieve control over the mind. Patanjali took the approach that matter and spirit needed to be separated to achieve such a state. Therefore, physical exercise formed only one of the eight limbs. Even then, the objective of the physical exercise was to prepare the body for prolonged meditation. The remaining pathways focused on a particular way of life, mental preparation or breathing. B.K.S. Iyengar provides a detailed study in his *Light on the Yoga Sutras of Patanjali* (2002) and there is a useful summary in his *Light on Yoga* (1991).

Hatha Yoga Pradipika (1400s)

The importance of asanas, physical training, was rekindled much later after Patanjali's approach. Hatha yoga, for example, is a particular system introduced in the fifteenth century in the scripture Hatha Yoga Pradipika. Hatha yoga was presented as a way of achieving Raja yoga through the physical preparation of the body ready for meditation. Through this realignment of focus, yoga then developed into a practice that made yoga practitioners focus on developing the body to make it immortal, rather than the spirit.

Yoga Today

By the 1960s yoga had been introduced into the West through an influx of Indian yoga teachers, following the movement of vegetarianism in the 1930s. Hatha yoga is the form that is most practised in the West, gaining far more popularity in the US than in Europe. Various forms of yoga have arisen over time due to the practices and teaching methods of particular instructors and their preferred focus and personal aspirations. When choosing which school of yoga to join, it is best to consider what your own aspirations are and then to find the appropriate yoga practice and instructor to fit that.

Your Pathway to Yoga

Students arrive at the decision to try yoga for a variety of reasons, ranging from mere curiosity or seeking relief from stress to a real desire for physical and spiritual development. Yoga practice requires much patience and perseverance but at the same time it should also be enjoyable and rewarding. Yoga is not a competitive sport. The objective should be personal development. You should not be disheartened by others who are more flexible than you and equally you should be encouraging to those less able.

By taking up yoga you take the first steps on your own very personal journey and that's where this book comes in. This work focuses on yoga training through physical exercises in order to improve flexibility, strength and balance. If that is the area on which you would like to focus then this text will complement your training.

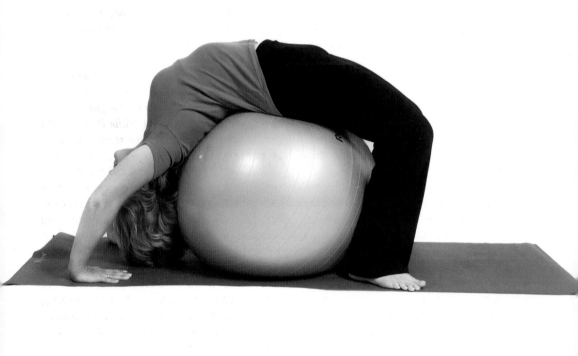

2   Guide for Beginners

The most important thing about training in yoga is that it will take much patience and perseverance before you start to see the benefits. When getting started, do not be too hard on yourself about your ability level. The stiffer you are, the more you have to benefit. Yoga is not a race or a competition. Your progress is only measured against how you are progressing from your own starting point. Do not judge yourself against fellow students. You must focus on your own development and give your body the time that it needs to improve.

Regular practice is the key to success in yoga, no matter where you are starting from. Do not be disheartened if you are not able to achieve complete poses. Use the preparation steps in this book to help you on your journey. Given time, you should be able to progress from one step to the next, eventually mastering the complete pose. There is much satisfaction to be gained from these very personal achievements, however large or small they are. This chapter will explain how you can use this book to:

- *Establish your range of motion*
- *Plan sessions to meet your development needs*
- *Modify exercises to suit your ability level*
- *Track your progress*

Safe training is the highest priority and so this chapter looks at the contraindications to training and provides some simple guidelines to help promote safe training. While it is possible to train in yoga without any specific requirements for equipment, you might make your training more comfortable through the use of equipment. Most students tend to use yoga mats as these provide both cushioning underneath the body when performing poses and frictional support to help them from slipping while holding poses. You may not always be able to control your training environment, but there are some considerations that can help enhance your enjoyment of your training through simple adjustments, such as adding relaxing music or ensuring that the space is clean, warm and airy.

Getting Started

Your Ability Level

Yoga is not a competitive sport. You do not need to have a certain level of flexibility in order to take part. Yoga practice is suitable for all levels of ability. Indeed, the stiffer you are, the more potential benefit you have to gain from such training. When joining a yoga class and starting training, do not be disheartened by people around you who may be more able. View them as sources of inspiration and allow them to show you the benefits that they have enjoyed.

Your current level of ability will be determined by many factors, including:

• What range of motion you commonly use
• What activities you are currently involved in
• What other activities you have been involved with in the past
• If you have had operations or injuries

Good yoga practice should indicate to you the areas where you are well developed and other areas that require more work. Do not shy away from what you learn about yourself. Instead, use this information to guide your training so that your body can become better balanced over time. You may be surprised to learn that you are perhaps more flexible on one side than the other. Or that you are able to do certain difficult poses that use certain parts of the body, but only simpler poses that use other parts. Whatever you learn, use these signs to encourage you to get yourself into better shape.

Your Range of Motion

The range of motion of your muscles is the range between the muscle being fully extended to that when it is fully contracted.

In order to maintain your current range of motion, you need to take your body through this full range regularly throughout the body. This will help you to maintain both the extensibility and the elasticity in the muscles. Without such regular training, the muscles will gradually shorten and this will alter the function of the joints and could also put undue stress on other parts of the body leading to injuries.

Through stretching and yoga exercises you can work towards maintaining and even improving your range of motion. As you work through the exercises in this book, you may well be surprised to find that your body can no longer perform movements that you could do when you were younger.

Your Development Plan

The exercises and poses given below (see Chapters 4 to 8) are presented using a step by step approach. These individual steps can give you an indication of the range of motion required for the various poses. Using these steps you can identify which step you can reach in any given exercise and use the progressive steps to track your progress. If you take a break in training, then you can also use the steps here to identify where, if anywhere, you have experienced a reduction in your range of motion.

Taking even a couple of weeks away from training can leave you feeling stiffer than normal, indicating the benefit you had been receiving through your training. It is for this reason that people generally become less flexible as they get older. If you attend classes containing a mix of age groups, you will be able to see some of the effects aging has on the range of motion. Children tend to be very flexible, easily performing exercises such as the lotus pose without effort. Similarly, older people may find that even some of the simple exercises presented as preparation exercises are difficult, for example, the neck and arm exercises. These observations can show just how much of an effect there can be if you do not train regularly.

To establish your range of motion with respect to each exercise, work your way through the exercises (see Chapters 4 to 8) and put a date against the exercises that you can already perform. You should also keep track of any imbalances you notice on one side compared to the other, and any muscles that you feel need more work, by keeping notes next to the pictures of each step. Use the anatomical diagrams to help you identify the muscle groups that you need to work on (see Chapter 3). Then, given time and practice, you can monitor your progress by putting dates against the more advanced steps as you achieve them. Through this process you will be able to track your progress and use this book to motivate you in your training.

This method will give a good indication of your ability level and also identify cases where you are unable to complete a particular pose. When this happens, you can instead focus your efforts on the preliminary steps to allow your body the time that it needs to develop. This method of tracking will indicate how quickly your muscles are able to develop their range of motion.

You can then use the session planner as a way of structuring training sessions to suit your development needs. Your development plan will not necessarily have time elements associated with it, as you will need to give your body the time it requires to develop the muscles. You can set yourself goals within specific exercises where you want to focus and which steps you wish to be able to achieve. You should then regularly review your plan to update your goals and adapt it according to how your body has progressed so far.

Putting Together Your Development Plan

1. Work through the exercises in this book putting a date against the steps that you can achieve comfortably.
2. Keep notes against the steps concerning things that you notice like imbalances, or which muscles or joints need particular work.
3. Use the anatomical diagrams (see Chapter 3) to help identify your development needs.
4. Add to your development needs any sport-specific training that you need.
5. Use the session planner (see Chapter 9) to create sample session plans.
6. Date the exercise steps in this book as you progress.
7. Review your development goals and plan regularly.

Practising Yoga

Training in yoga is not an easy option. To really reap the benefits, you must have patience and perseverance. Seeing improvement in your ability will be a slow, gradual and often surprising process. Do not expect just one or two lessons to show marked progress: it may take four or five before you begin to feel any improvement. Yoga training is not a race. You must allow your body the time it needs to develop and grow stronger.

• Practise regularly
• Make movements slowly and safely
• Don't go too far too quickly!

It is best to practise yoga regularly. Two to three times a week should certainly be enough to start to show you some benefits. Breaks in training will inevitably result in you feeling stiffer. With time, yoga will become something that merges more and more into your everyday life, affecting how you sit and how you feel when you move.

When starting in yoga, you may well find that there are few poses you can achieve completely and comfortably. This is not a problem. It only indicates that you must first work on the preparatory positions that will eventually enable you to achieve the full pose. This book can help show you how to get into each of the poses and these preparation steps are excellent places to stop and focus your training until you are comfortable enough to progress further. Too many students try to go too far too quickly. This will only result in pain and perhaps even injury, and it will not aid your training as it may mean that you want to, or even need to, take time out. You must be patient with your body.

Moving in and out of positions should be done slowly and safely. If you are unsure about how fast to move, then a useful indicator is to time your movements with your breathing, which should be deep and relaxed. To get the most out of your practice, you should feel a stretch in the muscles that you are working. This may feel slightly uncomfortable, but it should be a good discomfort, which means that your muscles are working at the right level. You should not feel pain. If you do begin to feel pain, then you must either come out of the pose or make the pose slightly easier for yourself by pulling back a little or even moving back to an earlier step. Pain and injury will not aid your training, only hinder it. When a particular pose has been mastered, it will become effortless and cause no discomfort.

Fitness

How fit you are is not just based on how fast and how far you can run or how much weight you can lift. There are many different elements to fitness.

If you are interested in improving your overall fitness, then a training regime that addresses most, if not all, the components of fitness is probably what you are looking for. In yoga, flexibility is not the only aspect of your fitness that can be developed. Poses often also require strength and an ability to balance. To master poses and maintain them for longer durations will sometimes require a combination of all three. Training can also help to develop your spatial awareness and your posture.

When working on a pose it is worth thinking about which element of your fitness is being developed. It won't necessarily be your flexibility. Indeed, your answer may even be different to that of another student.

The Components of Fitness

Flexibility	The range of movement around a joint
Strength	The capacity to exert maximal forces and to withstand fatigue
Balance	The state where forces acting on the body are distributed evenly
Stamina	The capacity of the body to sustain low level aerobic work with time
Speed	The capacity to move the whole body or limbs quickly
Agility	The capacity to change direction quickly
Power	The capacity to generate large amounts of force in short periods of time
Posture	The capacity of certain muscles to maintain efficient body alignment
Coordination	The ability to move body parts in the correct sequence

Some poses also test your strength and others also test your ability to balance. The focus of this book is on developing flexibility, strength and balance. Yoga poses can be performed in different ways in order to achieve different results. For this reason, having in the back of your mind what it is that you are trying to achieve through your practice will help to get the most out of your training.

Developing Flexibility

If your aim is to improve your flexibility, then you can start by first establishing your range of movement, as related to the particular exercise you are working on, and then work the body close to those limits. Once in position, hold the pose and give the muscles time to gently relax into the new position. This will help towards improving your flexibility. You should not at any stage need to work through pain. It takes time for the muscles to develop. Through regular practice, you should gradually begin to see improvements. These may not come all at once or be very noticeable at first, but over time you should be able to see the changes. Yoga stretches can be done statically or incorporated into movement. Different types of practice will have differing effects on how you develop and how fast you develop. There are several different types of stretching that can be applied during training (see Chapter 3). When working on poses, being aware of the type of stretching that you are using should help to reduce the risk of injury.

Developing Strength

Although developing strength may not be the first thing you might have thought yoga would require, once you start training you may well find that certain poses, even if they look simple, require a great deal of strength in order to be able to get into and then main-

tain them. As your training progresses, you should find that you can hold positions that require strength for longer and longer, and that perhaps they even begin to feel easier. You can challenge yourself by encouraging your body to stay in position for just a little longer each time. Yoga does not require any equipment or weights and so all the strength work that you do will be under your own body weight.

Developing Balance

Some exercises can look deceptively easy, particularly those that require balance. If you are lucky you may find that you are naturally good at balancing. Should you have difficulty in achieving any of the balancing poses, however, then it is better to focus on one of the preparatory steps instead until you are ready to progress through to the whole pose. Watching other students wobbling in their poses may also tend to make you feel unstable. Focusing your gaze on a steady point in front of you should help you to balance. Balancing with your eyes closed can be more difficult and so it is best to start with your eyes open before moving on. If you wish, you can even use a wall to give some support while you are working towards improving your balance, as this will help you to get into the pose first, rather than trying to do all things at once. Again, you should work towards holding the pose for longer in order to help improve your balance. It is better to hold a slightly easier position for a while than to hold a difficult position only momentarily.

Training Considerations

Safety

When you join a yoga class, you will find that the instructor will either get you to complete a health check form or will ask if you have any injuries or conditions that they should be aware of. It is important for the instructor to know whether you are fit to participate in the class. A good instructor should be mindful of your limitations and encourage appropriate modifications to practices to ensure that you are able to fully participate in the lesson.

Important

This book is intended to complement training done under the supervision of a trained instructor and is no substitute for a teacher.

The student must remember at all times, however, that a yoga instructor is not qualified to give medical advice. If students are unsure about certain injuries or conditions, and whether or not they should participate, then it is their responsibility to ensure that they get advice from appropriately qualified medical professionals. The most important thing is to ensure that you are training in a safe manner.

Training Tips

There are some basic guidelines that will make your training more comfortable and beneficial:

• Do not train immediately after a heavy meal
• Do not train on an empty stomach as your muscles work better when supplied with sufficient nutrients
• Do not practise after being out in the hot sun for several hours
• A short period of relaxation after practice is recommended

• If possible, bathe both before and after training to refresh yourself

Here are some tips to help you during training:

• Where a position is shown using one side of the body, your training should ensure that you practise on both sides.
• It is better to hold a slightly easier position for longer than to push your body into a difficult position that you can hold for only a few seconds.
• Pay attention to instructions, especially when they are regarding safety
• You should keep a bottle of water near you during training
• Sit out of any exercises that you are uncomfortable with for any reason
• Breathing must be comfortable and not restricted
• Try to breathe through the nose rather than the mouth

Steadying the Mind

The original objective of practising yoga was to steady the mind. When you are in a position, your focus should be on the present. Your mind should be clear of all other thoughts and concerns. Keeping your breathing deep and slow should help you to reach this state. Once in a position, try to relax and feel calm. Let the body do the work and let the mind have a rest.

Using the Eyes

Most exercises are best practised with the eyes open to start with, especially balancing and strengthening exercises. As time goes on and the poses come to you more easily and naturally, you can practise the poses with your eyes closed. By this stage you should have a better understanding of your alignment and be able to recognize when you have correctly achieved a pose.

Training in a Group

Although yoga training itself is very much an individual activity, it is much easier to be disciplined about regular training when with a group. Students often report that they find it difficult to motivate themselves to hold simple poses for any length of time when they are on their own, whereas in a group environment you will be encouraged and supported to keep going. Over time, it should become easier to incorporate simple exercises into everyday life, such as watching television while sitting cross-legged or using simple wrist and arm exercises when you feel stiff in the office or at work.

Working with a Partner

Although working with a partner can be beneficial, this book focuses on individual training as it is a much safer alternative. Due to the large variation in flexibility in individuals and also the unknown aspect of previous muscle injuries and trauma, as well as simple natural variations in individuals' skeletal and muscular structure, it is recommended that exercises are performed as an individual. Only the individual can tell when they have reached their maximum comfort levels and also when the stretch has gone too far and is causing them pain. Individual training allows constant monitoring and adjustment of the position. In addition, training alone raises your awareness levels so that you can begin to understand how your own body responds under such practice.

Training Contraindications

There a number of contraindications to training. If you have any pre-existing medical condition, you should seek advice from a medical professional before beginning any training regime. In particular, it is important to take note of the following:

- If you have high blood pressure, suffer from dizziness, have displacement of the retina or suffer from pus in the ears then avoid inverted poses and take extra care during yoga exercise
- Avoid compressive poses if they make you feel uncomfortable
- Avoid inverted poses during menstruation
- No undue stress should be felt in the head

In general, the best way to practise yoga is to do only the poses that you are comfortable with. If a certain pose is too difficult, then it is better to find an easier version that you can manage rather than place undue stress on your body. When training in a yoga class, do not feel under any pressure to try to 'keep up' with other students. Just sit out from any exercises that you do not wish to try. Yoga practice is not a competition. The most important thing is to train at your own pace and give your body the time that it needs to become comfortable with the poses.

When you are pregnant and after delivery, until you have fully recovered, it is best to obtain medical advice about taking part in yoga training. Many women find that the breathing and relaxation techniques learned through training in yoga and the ability to control the contraction and relaxation of muscles can be of great help during early labour contractions.

Sports Injuries

Many students take up training in yoga following a sporting or other injury. In these circumstances, it is again advisable to first seek medical advice on which type of exercises must be avoided. Many students of yoga have found that training can help to regain flexibility and strength in the affected regions. This process is gradual, however, and students will need to be patient in dealing with recovering from injuries.

Training Equipment

It is possible to train in yoga with a minimum of equipment. This suits many people as it is an activity that therefore requires little capital outlay in order to take part. However, depending on your ability level, you may feel that some of the following equipment would be helpful.

Clothing

There is no yoga uniform as such. Loose comfortable clothing is recommended and, depending on the climate where you are training, it is useful to have clothes that will keep you warm. For example, if you are training in a warm or even a hot environment, then shorts and a T-shirt or vest will probably be most appropriate. It is better that your training top is quite flexible but not very loose, as otherwise it can be quite uncomfortable when performing inverted exercises. Muscles are best kept warm during yoga training. This can be achieved by either increasing the temperature of your environment or by wearing appropriate and comfortable clothing.

Training Mats

Depending on the kind of floor that you are training on and also your level of flexibility, a towel or yoga training mat can be useful. For some poses, such as standing poses where the feet are quite far apart, a mat will provide frictional support and help you to reduce slipping during exercises. A towel is useful for defining your own training space and also making training more comfortable when the floor is not quite clean. Mats, on the other hand, are useful if you require some cushioning beneath you. This is particularly the case if you are training on a wooden or other solid floor. If you are training on carpet, then you may find that a training mat is not necessarily required, except for certain exercises. The main benefits of training mats is that they:

• Provide cushioning
• Define your training space
• Provide frictional support

When choosing a training mat you should consider the following factors:

• How will you transport it to and from where you train? Not all mats fold compactly and they can be cumbersome if you walk or cycle to your training location.
• How much cushioning do you feel you need? Training mats come in a variety of thicknesses. In general, the thicker mats will weigh more and be more cumbersome.
• Some mats give better friction support than others. If you can, it's best to try out a variety with your bare feet and see which one best supports you from slipping.

Blocks

Yoga training blocks are available in various shapes and sizes. They can be useful for beginners in particular. For example, they can be used for providing support during exercises that require resting the hands on the ground and where the student cannot reach. Having several different sizes of blocks at your disposal will mean that you can use them as appropriate to the exercise to provide you with the right level of support. Balancing exercises are another example where students find blocks useful, particularly if they cannot reach the ground with their hands on their own accord.

Blocks can also be great for providing support to students that have trouble sitting comfortably on the ground cross-legged. Raising the student slightly off the

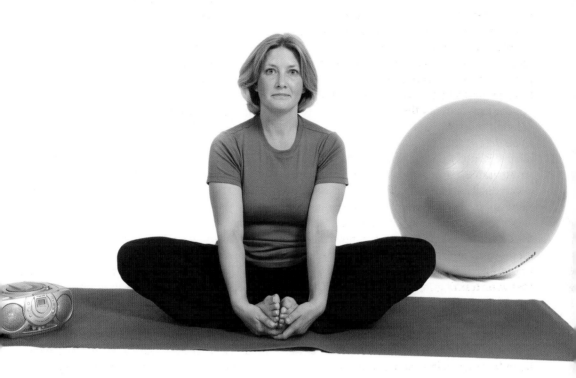

Yoga training equipment.

ground relieves the stress in the ankles and can make training a lot more enjoyable until sufficient flexibility levels are reached that will allow training without blocks.

Straps

Straps again are useful particularly if, for example, you cannot reach your toes when attempting the seated forward bend position (posterior pose). The strap can then be used to enable correct back positioning even though your hands cannot reach your feet. This way you can still focus on bending forward from your hip rather than from your back and your neck. This makes training a lot safer if

you have limited flexibility. Just hold each end of the strap in each of your hands and wrap the middle of the strap around your feet. You can then adjust the strap to ensure that you get a stretch during the exercise.

Ball

An inflatable yoga ball can be used to provide support when performing exercises like the wheel pose, where your back is arched and your hands and feet are supporting your weight. This will enable you to relieve some of the pressure of the exercise by resting your back on the ball. It will also take some of the weight off your arms.

29

Music

Not all yoga classes use music but it can be a great way to relax the mind and let the body focus on the exercise. Music with no singing but a simple rhythmic and repetitive melody is particularly recommended. When training outside, try to choose your location based on the sounds around you. For example, training on the beach near the water can be really calming as you hear the waves repeatedly breaking on the shore. Sounds of nature are also soothing to listen to during training, for example birds and forest sounds. A small portable stereo can be ideal for providing background music to complement your training.

Hydration

Depending on how demanding your yoga session is, it can be useful to keep some water with you in training. This is especially so if you are in a warm or even hot environment and you are working on exercises that use your muscles intensely, making you feel hot and sweaty or even out of breath.

Training Environment

An important part of enjoying yoga is being comfortable in the environment within which you train. The ideal requirements are for the space to be clean, free from distraction and comfortably warm. While you may not necessarily have control over your training location, here are some considerations for choosing and preparing a training environment.

Temperature

Ideally you want to train where the temperature is comfortable enough for you to wear a T-shirt or vest without getting cold. In general, the warmer the environment the better, as your muscles develop the best under these conditions. You may generally feel that you have achieved much more through your training when it is warmer. It is usual for students to see much greater improvements in flexibility when training over the summer than in the winter.

Floor

Ideally the training floor should be clean and the room should have good light and air. A wooden floor is great for training on but will most probably require the use of mats to make training comfortable. If you train on a carpeted floor, then you may find it difficult to do balancing exercises without the aid of a mat.

Mirrors

Training in front of a mirror can make it easier to judge whether you are aligned or not. This kind of observation and self-correction will stand you in good stead as it will make it easier for your body to naturally get into poses correctly with practice and you will be more aware of when you are not correctly aligned.

The View

Training in a pleasant and relaxing looking environment free from distraction will help you to stay focused on your training and also enhance your enjoyment. Training in a dark, gloomy room will tend to make it more difficult to feel relaxed and get the most out of your training.

Training Outdoors

Yoga training is not restricted to being indoors. Training outdoors brings a whole new element to your yoga training. The fact that yoga practice requires little or no equipment makes it an ideal activity for outdoors. Whether during your holidays or just incorporating a few exercises into your work life, it will bring the benefits of yoga to other aspects of your life.

The first requirements of finding a suitable outdoor space in which to train are that it must be safe from any dangerous objects on the ground, the climate appropriate and there should be sufficient protection from the sun and wind. Many yoga students love to train on the beach. This can be a wonderful experience if the temperature is not too hot and you have the sound of the waves lapping on the shore in the background. A calm and peaceful environment is ideal. Training on the grass in the garden or in a park can also be great fun.

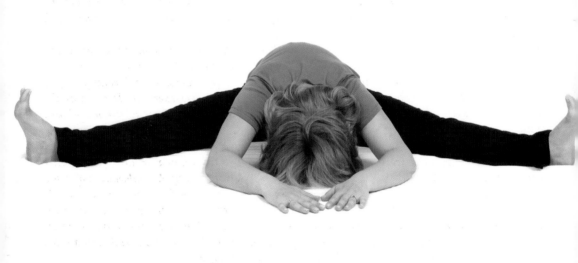

3 Your Body and Yoga

Although training in yoga does not require a detailed understanding of how the muscles and the joints work, it certainly can be useful to have some basic understanding, as this will increase your appreciation for your training. Many students often ask about what exercises will help certain muscles and also which muscles are being worked in any given exercise. This chapter will help you to identify the parts of the body that you are developing through your training and in any particular exercise. In addition, knowing where the muscles are, how they connect to the bones and how each of the major joints work can give you a better indication of the potential to be gained from each exercise.

Yoga instructors should usually check your alignment and posture, so ensuring that you are working the correct muscles for that particular exercise. If, for example, your leg is slightly rotated when it should be straight, then you will be working the leg muscles in a different way to what the pose intended. Sometimes incorrect alignment over many repetitions of an exercise may cause discomfort and even increase the risk of injuries.

This chapter presents a basic introduction to both the skeletal and the muscular system in relation to the stretching and contracting of muscles during yoga exercises. It explains the different stages of muscle contraction and how to describe movement. There are number of different ways to stretch: static, active, PNF (proprioceptive neuromuscular facilitation) and ballistic stretching. A combination of static and PNF stretching is considered to provide the safest method of training. During training you may well feel muscle fatigue and soreness. This chapter looks at the potential mechanisms behind these effects.

Understanding the Human Body and Movement

The most common questions that students ask tend to be regarding which muscles they are working and what they could potentially achieve. Having an understanding of how the skeletal and muscular systems work can help you to get more out of your yoga practice and answer these questions for you, as and when they arise. It can enable you to identify which of the major muscle groups you are working through the various exercises. You may not always feel the same muscles working as another individual while doing the same exercises, as it can depend on your ability level and your developmental requirements as to where your body is actively working.

A basic understanding of the human body and movement will give you an appreciation of the way that the different joints work and what you can expect of them. The right terminology will help you to better communicate with your instructor and fellow students as well as raising your own awareness of how your body functions.

The Skeletal System

From a yoga perspective, the main function of the skeletal system is to provide the anchor points for the muscles to pull on in order to create movement. The bones of the skeleton are joined by ligaments, thus forming the joints of the body. The skeleton is a hard framework of 206 bones that support and protect the muscles and organs of the human body. It is divided into two parts:

• The axial skeleton: this supports the head, neck and trunk. It consists of the skull, the vertebral column, the ribs and the sternum.

• The appendicular skeleton: this supports the appendages or limbs and attaches them to the rest of the body. It consists of the shoulder girdle, the upper limbs, the pelvic girdle and the lower limbs.

The shoulder girdle comprises the clavicle, the scapula and the humerus. The pelvic girdle comprises the innominate bones, the sacrum, the femur, the coccyx and the symphysis pubis. The wrist comprises eight carpal bones and the hand comprises five metacarpal bones. The fingers are composed of fourteen phalanges in each hand, two in the thumb and three in each of the fingers. The ankle and the foot comprise seven tarsals and five metatarsals. The toes are composed of fourteen phalanges in each foot, two in the big toe and three in each of the other toes.

From a yoga perspective, the main functions of the skeleton are:

• Allows and enables movement
• Forms joints which are essential for the movement of the body
• Provides attachment for muscles that move the joints

Defining Movement

All muscles work by contraction but each muscle performs a specific movement in order to move the body. It can be useful to use consistent terminology for describing movement and it should make it easier for you to communicate more effectively with fellow students and your instructor. There are a number of different actions and these are shown in the diagram on page 36.

Joint Types

Joints are the body's hinges and there are three types: fixed, slightly moveable and freely moveable. The pelvic girdle is an

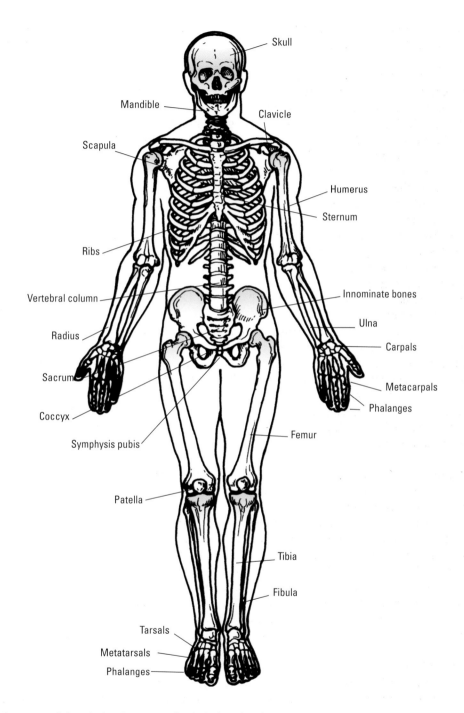

The main parts of the skeletal system that are involved
in yoga training.

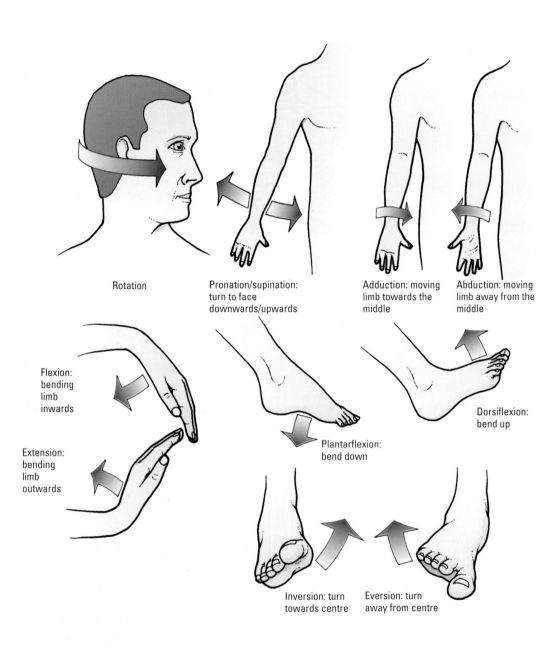

Rotation

Pronation/supination: turn to face downwards/upwards

Adduction: moving limb towards the middle

Abduction: moving limb away from the middle

Flexion: bending limb inwards

Extension: bending limb outwards

Plantarflexion: bend down

Dorsiflexion: bend up

Inversion: turn towards centre

Eversion: turn away from centre

Terminology for describing movement.

Joint Types

Slightly moveable joint

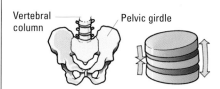

Also known as a cartilaginous joint. It moves by the compression of the cartilage between the bones, for example in the vertebral column.

Ball and socket joint

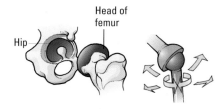

The most moveable of all joints. Allows flexion, extension, adduction, abduction, rotation and circumduction, for example, in the shoulder and hip joints.

Hinge joint

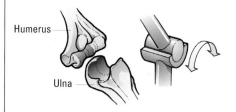

Allows movement in one direction or plane only. Movements are flexion and extension in, for example, the elbow, the knee, the ankle, the joints between the phalanges of the fingers and the toes.

Gliding joint

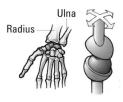

Allows bones to glide over each other, for example between the tarsals and between the carpals.

Pivot joint

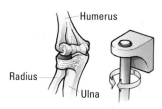

Allows movement around one axis only. This is a rotary movement, for example, in the radius and the ulna joint.

Saddle joint

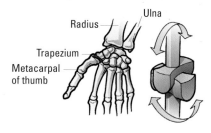

Allows movement around two axes, allowing flexion, extension, adduction, abduction, circumduction, for example in the wrist.

example of a fixed joint, so it allows no movement. There are then six types of moveable joints: slightly moveable joint, ball and socket joint, hinge joint, gliding joint, pivot joint and saddle joint.

The Main Joints Used in Yoga and Their Movements

- The hip is a ball and socket joint and can bend towards and straighten away from the body and also rotate.
- The shoulder is a ball and socket joint and can bend towards and straighten away from the body and also rotate.
- The radius-ulnar is a pivot joint and can rotate.
- The elbow is a hinge joint and can bend and straighten.
- The knee is a hinge joint and can bend and straighten.
- The ankle is a hinge joint and can bend and straighten.
- The wrist is a saddle joint and can bend towards and straighten away from the body and also rotate.

The Muscular System

A muscle is a group of specialized elastic tissues. Muscle typically makes up to around 23 per cent of a woman's body weight and around 40 per cent of a man's body weight. Muscles consist of bundles of fibres attached to bones at each end by tendons. Muscles shorten as a result of receiving signals from the brain and the spinal cord, which travel to the muscles via the nerves. The shortening of the muscles brings about movement of the skeleton. Muscle tissue is bound together in bundles and contained in a sheath, sometimes called the fascia, the end of which extends to form a tendon that attaches the muscle to other parts of the body. A muscle's function is to contract and by doing so to start a movement in the surrounding structures, the ligaments, the tendons and eventually the bones. The muscle then shortens, becoming fatter in the centre.

Muscles never work alone. Any movement results from the actions of several muscles. In general, muscles work in pairs. Each pair contains an antagonist (the relaxing muscle) and the agonist (the contracting muscle). They must both relax and contract equally to ensure smooth movement.

Muscles get their energy from the oxygen and nutrients supplied by the blood. Blood is also responsible for carrying away any waste products such as urea and lactic acid. A muscle's ability to contract is affected by the following factors:

- Energy available
- Strength of the stimulus from the nerve
- Time the muscle has been contracting
- Adequate blood supply bringing sufficient oxygen and nutrients
- Strength of the inhibitory nerve system
- Temperature of the muscle (warmth increases the response)
- Presence of waste products like lactic acid

Stages of Muscle Contraction

In normal healthy muscles, there will always be a few muscle fibres contracting at any one time, even during sleep. This action gives normal posture to the body. This is called muscle tone and it is the slight degree of contraction by some fibres while others are relaxing. Relaxation is when there is a reduction in the number of fibres contracting at any one time. This can be achieved by conscious effort and assisted relaxation.

The Major Muscle Groups

Possibly the most useful information for yoga practitioners, and certainly forming one of the most commonly asked questions, is what muscles are students working when in any given yoga pose. Understanding the where-abouts of the major muscle groups in the body can greatly help you. It will give you the information you need to identify which muscles you are using during the stretches of the yoga poses for yourself, through being aware of where you feel the stretch. It will also give you an appreciation of the reasons for aligning the body in a particular way during the poses, as it is through this process that you can ensure that the right muscles are being engaged in any given pose. It will also help you to communicate clearly with others about your personal goals.

The muscle group known as the quadriceps (full name quadriceps femoris) is a composite muscle consisting of the rectus femoris, the vastus lateralis, the vastus medialis and the vastus intermedius. The vastus intermedius is located between the vastus lateralis and the vastus medialis, and is below the rectus femoris. Similarly, the hamstrings are also a group of muscles: the biceps femoris, the semi-tendinous and the semi-membranosus.

The inside leg muscles that are used for performing exercises like the angle pose and the side splits are the hip adductors: the adductor brevis, the adductor longus and the adductor magnus. All three of these orig-inate on the pubis. The adductor brevis is situated behind the adductor longus.

Types of Stretching

Stretching is an important part of any fitness regime and can help to reduce muscle fatigue and injuries. Yoga exercises already form many of the stretching exercises that are commonly seen in other sports. There are a number of different ways to work the muscles during stretching exercises and it can be helpful to be able to distinguish between them. Yoga poses can be performed by using each of these different stretching techniques. However, the benefits from each will be different.

Static Stretching

This involves taking a limb to the point at which tightness is felt and then holding this position. This is the sort of stretching that is mostly used in yoga. Once the muscle is held under tension for some time, it will gradually

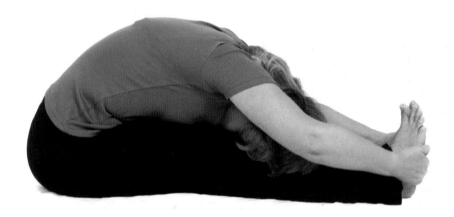

Example of static stretching: holding the posterior pose.

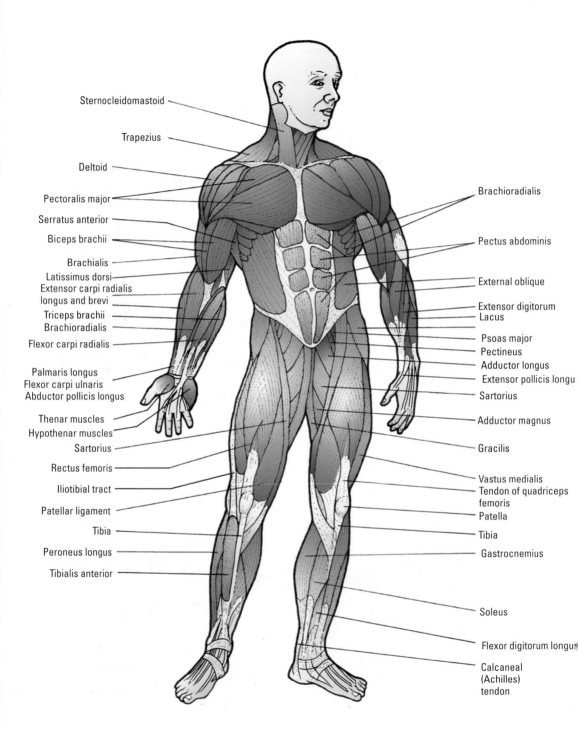

Sternocleidomastoid

Trapezius

Deltoid

Pectoralis major

Serratus anterior

Biceps brachii

Brachialis

Latissimus dorsi
Extensor carpi radialis
longus and brevi

Triceps brachii
Brachioradialis

Flexor carpi radialis

Palmaris longus
Flexor carpi ulnaris
Abductor pollicis longus

Thenar muscles
Hypothenar muscles

Sartorius

Rectus femoris

Iliotibial tract

Patellar ligament

Tibia

Peroneus longus

Tibialis anterior

Brachioradialis

Pectus abdominis

External oblique

Extensor digitorum
Lacus

Psoas major
Pectineus
Adductor longus
Extensor pollicis longu

Sartorius

Adductor magnus

Gracilis

Vastus medialis
Tendon of quadriceps
femoris
Patella

Tibia

Gastrocnemius

Soleus

Flexor digitorum longu

Calcaneal
(Achilles)
tendon

The major muscle groups at the front (anterior) of the body.

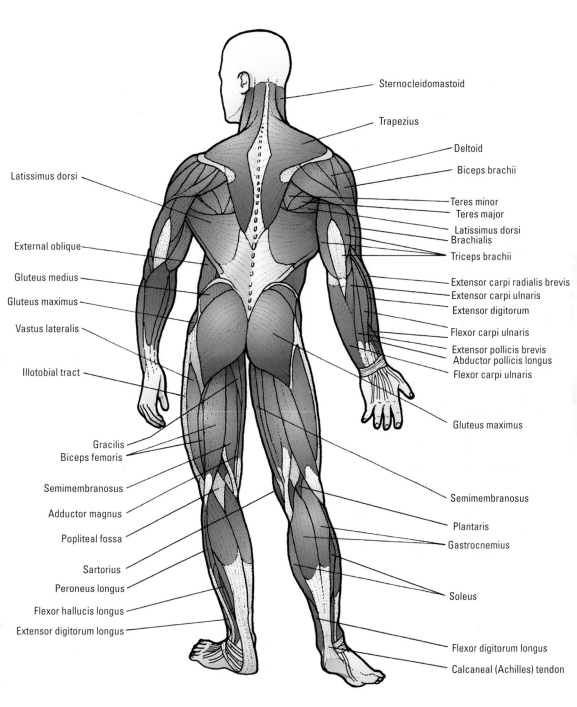

Sternocleidomastoid

Trapezius

Deltoid

Biceps brachii

Latissimus dorsi

Teres minor
Teres major
Latissimus dorsi
Brachialis
Triceps brachii

External oblique

Gluteus medius

Gluteus maximus

Vastus lateralis

Extensor carpi radialis brevis
Extensor carpi ulnaris
Extensor digitorum

Flexor carpi ulnaris

Extensor pollicis brevis
Abductor pollicis longus
Flexor carpi ulnaris

Illotobial tract

Gluteus maximus

Gracilis
Biceps femoris

Semimembranosus

Adductor magnus

Semimembranosus

Popliteal fossa

Plantaris
Gastrocnemius

Sartorius

Peroneus longus

Flexor hallucis longus

Soleus

Extensor digitorum longus

Flexor digitorum longus

Calcaneal (Achilles) tendon

The major muscle groups at the back (posterior) of the body.

elongate and relax. Since this position will need to be held for some time, it is important that you start off in a comfortable position. From this position, it is best to release the muscle tension in a slow and controlled manner. Static stretching is considered the safest method of stretching and it is recommended for use in the yoga positions in this book. Further information is available in Christopher Norris's *The Complete Guide to Stretching* (2001). Focusing on breathing at this stage can help you to relax the muscle even further. Through repeated practice and training, the muscle will gradually allow greater ranges of motion.

Active Stretching

This involves working two sets of muscle groups together. The agonist is the muscle or muscle group that contracts and the antagonist is the muscle or muscle group that stretches. Active stretching is where you get one muscle to contract to its full range, while requiring the antagonist to stretch to its full range. This is the type of

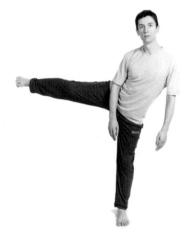

Step 2. Raise your rear leg to the side, while keeping your knee locked. Keep your upper body relaxed and in the same position.

stretching that is used in most sports for developing both flexibility and strength at the same time. Such an action requires good control over the movement and so it also develops skill. Active stretching is very common in the martial arts and ballet. An example of active stretching is shown below, where steps one to three would be completed in one smooth action.

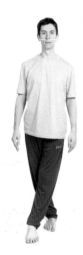

Step 1. Start with one foot in front of the other and crossed over.

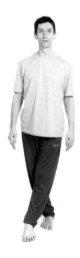

Step 3. Return your raised leg back to its starting position.

PNF Stretching

PNF (proprioceptive neuromuscular facilitation) stretching was developed by physiotherapists for the treatment of patients who had suffered strokes. It involves a series of movements designed to get the maximum out of a muscle using primitive muscle reflexes. The first technique is called contract-relax. Here the student must first contract the muscle to be stretched for ten to twenty seconds, using static stretching, followed by relaxing it and then repeating. This will help to increase the range of motion. This can be demonstrated using ankle flexion. Following steps one through to two gives an example of PNF contract-relax stretching.

The other method is called contract-relax-agonist-contract-relax. Here you start with the contract-relax process as above and then you contract and relax the opposing muscle. This gives the additional benefit of strengthening the muscle group that controls the full range of motion, so ensuring that any imbalances in muscle development are minimized. Following steps one through to four gives an example of PNF contract-relax-agonist-contract-relax stretching.

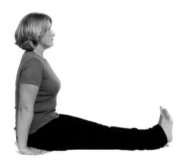

Step 1. Contract – Start by sitting with both of your legs together in front of you and one hip width apart. Then pull both of your feet in by bending at the ankle.

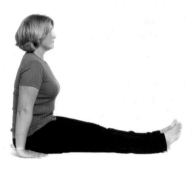

Step 2. Relax – Relax both of your feet into a natural position.

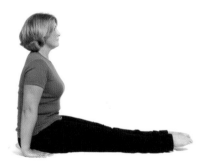

Step 3. Agonist contract – Point your feet forwards as far as possible.

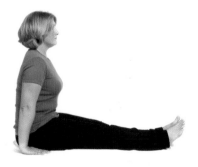

Step 4. Relax – Relax both of your feet back into a natural position.

Ballistic Stretching

This is considered the most unsafe form of stretching and so it is important that students are aware of its dangers. It involves moving the muscle to its maximum range and then repeating small bounces in order to try and achieve a greater stretch. This can be dangerous because it can make it impossible to control the movement and to stop before the muscle is overstretched. Repeatedly overstretching the muscle can lead to multiple small tears in the muscle tissue. This scar tissue can then build up over many years and can alter the mechanics of the joint altogether and also lead to other injuries. Such stretching can indeed have the opposite of the desired effect by actually decreasing flexibility. This is due to the stretch reflex action of the muscle, where a rapid stretch will cause the muscles to contract.

However, such stretching does not always result in injuries. Examples of this are found in ballet and the martial arts, where movements quite often use the full range of motion. When the actions are performed slowly and under control, then they are active stretches. If these actions are performed explosively and fast, however, then they become ballistic in nature. Since these students have trained in such movement, it is believed that their stretch reflex action is reset so that it does not actually occur as fast as the actual movement does. Inexperienced students should not attempt any ballistic stretching as the risk of injury is much higher.

Students suffering from injuries from ballistic stretching will need to train to regain both strength and flexibility gradually through other methods of stretching, namely static, active and PNF stretching.

Muscle Fatigue and Soreness

Yoga poses can work the muscles intensely and it is not uncommon for students to feel discomfort in their muscles. You may experience muscle fatigue and soreness at some point in your training and so it can be helpful to be able to identify it and also to understand the possible mechanisms that can lead to it.

When stimulated, a muscle will need oxygen and fuel. Muscles burn glucose and fats by combining them with oxygen from the blood. Muscles that are repeatedly contracting and relaxing need a lot of energy and this is why strenuous exercise causes rapid breathing, leading to breathlessness. If your muscle continues to contract without enough rest, your muscle will run out of oxygen and a by-product of this deficiency, lactic acid, will build up. This acid causes a burning sensation in the muscle. The muscle will then begin to quiver and will soon stop contracting. You will feel stiffness and pain in the affected muscle. The muscle will not work properly until it can remove the lactic acid. It will need a fresh supply of oxygen for this and you will need to slow down. This process is muscle fatigue.

The rate of onset of muscle fatigue often determines who will be the most easily frustrated when attempting to become physically fit. Fatigue is a complex phenomena that may have many different causes. It could lie in the nervous system, the muscular system or some combination of the two.

Although certain kinds of strenuous efforts are associated with muscle pain during the exercise period, muscle soreness often develops some hours or even days after the exertion. The soreness, which begins as fatigue, results from heavy contractions, especially those that have a large static component, and is thought to be caused by an inadequate blood flow to the working muscles. This deprives the muscles of oxygen and fails to wash 'pain substances' out of the muscles. There are several products of contraction that could build up in the muscles or tissue fluid surrounding the muscles and cause pain by stimulating nerve endings in the muscle or connective tissue within the muscle. Experiments have shown that lactic acid and potassium, for example, can cause local pain when they are injected into a muscle.

Possible Causes of Muscle Fatigue

The mechanism behind muscle soreness and fatigue is not yet well understood, however a number of hypotheses are presented in detail in David Lamb's *Physiology of Exercise* (1984). These include:

• Lactic acid accumulation hypothesis: Lactic acid accumulates to a greater extent in more intensive types of exercise and that more intensive exercise causes the greatest delayed muscle soreness.
• Muscle spasm hypothesis: Strenuous contractions cause a reduction in blood flow to the working muscles. This triggers the release of pain substances out of the muscle fibres into the tissue fluid where they stimulate the nerve endings. The pain receptors then cause reflex spastic contractions of the painful muscle fibres to further reduce blood flow and thus create a pain cycle.

• Tissue damage hypothesis: Free nerve endings are stimulated by swelling of the muscle tissue after microscopic damage to a few muscle fibres or their surrounding connective tissue.

Reducing Muscle Soreness

Soreness is more common after relatively intense muscle contractions. Soreness is also more common in those who are undertaking an exercise programme after a long period of inactivity. Therefore, it is better to start off with light activity and then gradually build it up. This will allow the muscle fibres to become toughened and adaptive to the training.

Muscle Cramps

Muscle cramps are thought to be caused by salt imbalances in the fluids surrounding the muscle fibres. For example, a disruption in the normal relationships between sodium, potassium and chloride concentrations inside and outside the muscle fibres can cause spastic contractions. The mechanism behind muscle cramps is not yet clearly understood.

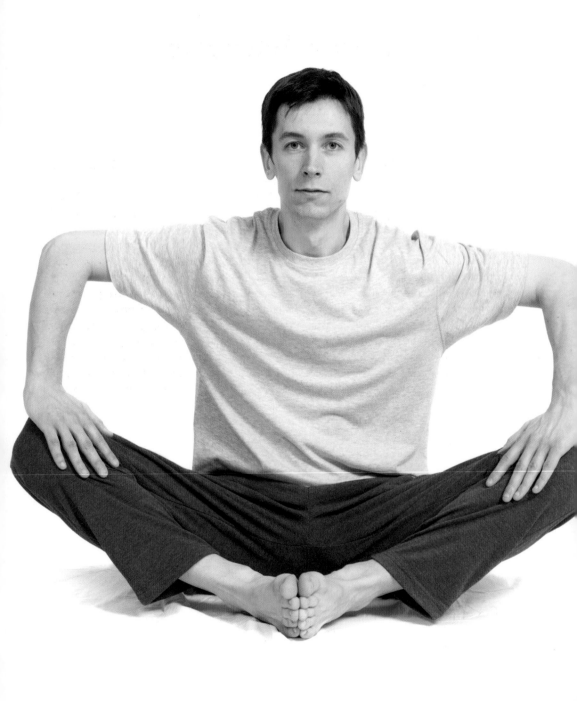

4   Preparation Exercises

This chapter presents a selection of simple exercises that can be used to prepare for a yoga lesson, for example, flexing the knees, shaking off the arms and legs, or rotating the ankles and wrists. These should help you to feel ready and relaxed going into the session. These light exercises can also be used in between yoga poses during the session as a way of reducing any stiffness that has built up. This can help you to become refreshed before the next pose. Simple preparation exercises can then be used to help bring the focus of your mind into the training and help you to relax, while also performing a light workout. Examples of these include gentle upper body exercises that work the wrists, arms and back.

There are a number of different ways to sit and these various sitting positions can be combined with the upper body exercises in this chapter to give you a light workout going into the session. You can also add deep and slow breathing during these exercises and it should leave you feeling refreshed and ready for some more challenging poses. Over time, the exercises in this chapter should help you to develop and maintain a good range of motion, particularly in the upper body. Many of these exercises may look easy, and yet many students find them very difficult. Give them a go and see how you get on.

Preparing the Body for Training

Shaking off the limbs, flexing the knees and rotating the ankles and wrists are all simple exercises that are a great way to get ready for training. They are best performed by keeping the body relaxed, muscles loose and the movements gentle. These exercises should feel refreshing and energizing and so they are also useful for loosening up between yoga poses or at the end of a session.

Shake Off

This simple yet effective exercise can be used at any time before, after or even during training. It can help to relieve any stiffness in the body, particularly in the arms and legs. Even a few seconds of this exercise can leave you feeling refreshed. During training, if you have been holding any pose for an extended time, then this exercise will help you to feel energized again before moving onto the next pose. The more demanding the pose attempted and the longer that it is held for, the more useful this exercise is.

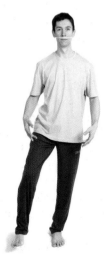

Stand with your legs a hip-width apart. Relax your hands, feet and shoulders. Then gently shake off your arms and legs.

Flex the Knees

This is another simple exercise that is useful for when your legs feel stiff or you feel any soreness building up behind the knees during training. The latter may happen, for example, while holding a seated forward bend position. You may also feel soreness around the knees when you are using the hip adductors, for example during the angle pose. A gentle flexing and straightening of the legs at the knees can help you to quickly relieve this and refresh the legs. You can perform this exercise right after coming out of any yoga pose where you feel that it will benefit you. Continue this exercise for as long as you feel necessary in order to reduce the soreness.

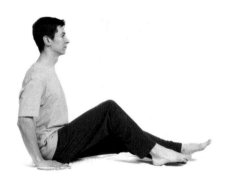

Sit with your legs a hip-width apart and straight out in front of you. Place your palms on the ground in line with your hips. Keep your upper body and feet relaxed and your shoulders down. Then alternately lift and lower your knees, gently bending and straightening in succession. Make the movement smooth and keep the muscles in your legs as relaxed as possible.

Ankle Rotation

This simple ankle rotation exercise can help to relieve stiffness and soreness in the ankles. It is also beneficial when releasing from poses that require bending at the ankle, such as the hero pose, the easy pose and even the more difficult lotus pose. If you find that you generally have quite stiff ankles, then this exercise should be a welcome release.

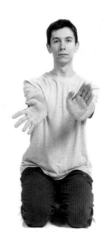

Start in a comfortable sitting position of your choice. Rotate around both of your wrists. Keep your shoulders relaxed and down.

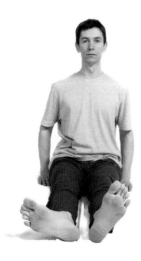

Sit with your legs comfortably apart and straight out in front of you. Place your palms on the ground in line with your hips. Keep your upper body and legs relaxed and your shoulders down. Rotate around both of your ankles.

Wrist Rotation

This wrist rotation exercise is similar to the ankle rotation. It can help to relieve stiffness and soreness in the wrists. It is also beneficial when releasing from poses that require bending at the wrists and taking weight onto the hands, such as the downward dog pose, the plank pose and the cobra pose. Since all of the aforementioned poses require much weight to be supported by the hands, the longer they are held the more you may feel your wrists become tired and stiff. Just performing this simple exercise can help to refresh them.

Sitting Positions

Sitting on the floor should feel natural and comfortable, but if you have become too used to sitting in a chair then this may not be the case. If you rarely sit on the floor, you may find the exercises in this section difficult or even impossible. However, if you are used to being seated on the floor, then you may find them quite simple. Even though you may have been able to sit on the floor comfortably for a long time when you were young, you may find that you are no longer able to now you are older. If this is the case, it may come as quite a surprise. This alone gives many students enough of a motivation to pursue yoga training in order to get back the ability that they know they used to have. If this is the case for you, then remember that you should use this to drive your training forwards and not as an excuse to give up.

A number of different sitting positions are shown here and you may find some easy and some impossible. They are presented in the general order of difficulty based on observations in class. It is better to work on a position that is slightly less challenging to get into, but more challenging to hold for a short period, say a few minutes. You can then work on building up the ability to remain comfortable in these positions for increasing amounts of time.

Stay seated in a particular pose for only as long as is comfortable. Feel free to change to a different sitting position to give your body a chance to recover and also then to engage other muscles. Some students find sitting cross-legged or kneeling impossible. In this case, it is advisable to start by sitting with the legs straight out in front of you and then slowly work to improve the ability to sit in different positions. The following tips are applicable to all of the sitting positions:

• Keep your back upright and straight.
• Rest your hands lightly on your knees or palms on the ground either side of your hips, as appropriate. Do not rest them behind you.
• Keep your shoulders relaxed and down.

You can also practise breathing slowly and deeply while in these various sitting positions. Try to take your mind off your body and let the muscles relax into the pose, while you focus on your breathing. Make sure that you make use of the full extent of your lungs. This may require some conscious effort to begin with, but given time this will become much easier and relaxing with practice.

These different sitting positions can be used effectively with other exercises that work only the upper body, for example the wrist and arm exercises described later in this chapter.

Staff Pose

The most basic sitting position is with your legs stretched out straight in front of you.

This simple exercise helps to raise your awareness of how you sit and your overall posture. Many yoga poses use this pose as a starting position and then work on moving the rest of the body into the correct position. Make sure that your back is straight and that your knees are not bent. Do not let your hands rest on the floor behind you. Instead, place the hands lightly on your legs or in front of you. This will help to ensure that you keep your back straight and upright and remain balanced. Varying the position of the feet will vary the muscles that are engaged during this stretch. For example, if you pull your feet back then you will engage the hamstrings and the calves. If you point the feet, then you will feel the muscles on the front of the legs working. The further apart you push your feet, the more you will engage the hip adductors.

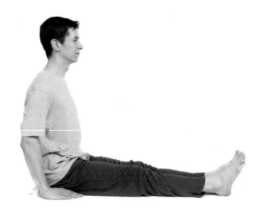

Sit with both legs straight out in front and your knees, heels and big toes touching. Push the back of your knees into the ground and do not let your legs rotate outwards. Place your palms flat on the ground either side of your hips and with your fingers pointing forwards. Keep your back straight and your shoulders down and pushed back slightly so that your chest is opened up. Push your pelvis slightly forward and bring your navel in slightly towards your spine. Hold your gaze parallel to the floor.

Angle Pose

The angle pose builds on the staff pose by separating the legs. This pose works the muscles on the inside of the legs and also helps to open up the hips. The wider the angle that your legs form, the greater your flexibility in performing this exercise. This again is a basic pose that is used as a starting position for more advanced yoga poses.

This exercise is particularly useful if you are training to improve your flexibility in order to achieve the side splits. Advanced students are able to get close to 180 degrees wide on this exercise. This ability will enable you to do more advanced poses as it opens the hip as well as developing good flexibility in the hip adductors. Students generally find sitting in this position fairly comfortable. The challenge is in getting the legs as wide apart as possible. If you feel soreness around the inside of the knees during this exercise, then you can use the flexing of the knees exercise to relieve some of this.

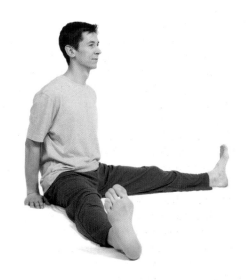

Step 2. Move your legs apart while keeping your knees locked. Aim to widen your legs to as far apart as you are comfortable and then hold. Push the back of your knees into the ground and do not let your legs rotate outwards. Keep your back straight and your shoulders down and pushed back slightly so that your chest is opened up. Push your pelvis slightly forward. Hold your gaze parallel to the floor. Ensure that the feet are pulled back so that the toes are pointing upwards.

Hero Pose

This is a great example of a position that looks simple and yet can be very challenging. In this basic kneeling position, you have your back straight and your bottom resting firmly between your feet and on the ground. Again, do not rest your hands on the ground behind you. It is best to rest them lightly on your knees. This exercise works your quadriceps and your knee and ankle joints. You may feel stiff around the joints when you come out of this position. In which case, the knee flexing and ankle rotation exercises are useful here. If you find this position difficult, then think about where you can feel the stretch the most, as this will indicate where you need to focus your development efforts.

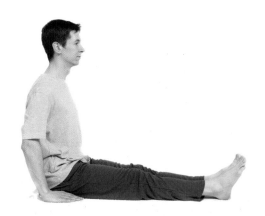

Step 1. Start in the staff pose.

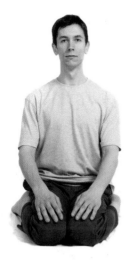

If you find sitting like this with the feet either side of your body difficult, then you could try the following variants, which are slightly easier. The first variant is the same kneeling position, but this time both feet are tucked underneath and the feet are overlapping. In the second variant, the feet are apart but still directly below the body and the bottom rests on top of the feet.

If you are starting with these simpler positions, then you will probably feel your ankles and knees doing quite a bit of the work. And so, you may find that it is uncomfortable sitting in these positions for very long. Regular practice should make it easier for you to begin to get more comfortable for longer.

Kneel with your feet either side of you, your hands resting lightly on the knees and your bottom touching the ground between your feet. The tops of your feet should be in contact with the ground and your toes should be pointing backwards. Your thighs should be parallel. Keep your back straight and your shoulders down and pushed back slightly so that your chest is opened up. Push your pelvis slightly forward. Hold your gaze parallel to the floor.

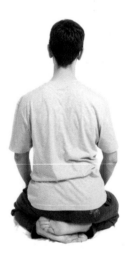

Variant 1: Feet overlapping. Place one foot on top of the other, with the toes pointing out to either side.

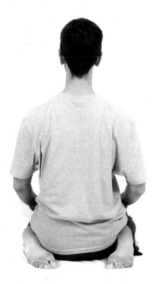

Rear view of the hero pose.

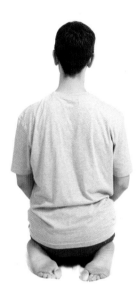
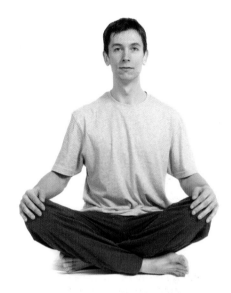

Variant 2: Feet slightly apart. Keep your feet a hip-width apart and directly underneath your bottom. Your toes should point backwards and your upper body weight should be supported on your heels.

Easy Pose

Sitting cross-legged on the ground is a very natural way to sit. This is called the easy pose. It should be possible to sit comfortably like this for extended periods of time. If you find that you are only comfortable for a few minutes, then you could practise sitting in this position and gradually increase the amount of time that you can manage. Sitting in the easy pose is the starting point to working towards the difficult lotus position, which is commonly associated with yoga and meditation. You should practise this pose on both sides, so that each foot has a turn at resting on top.

Some may find this position uncomfortable or even impossible. With training the body will get used to sitting on the floor in this way. Eventually, sitting in these positions will become effortless.

Sit cross-legged with both feet tucked underneath. The sides of the feet should touch the ground rather than the tops of your feet. Rest your hands lightly on your knees and keep your upper body relaxed. Keep your back straight and your shoulders down and pushed back slightly so that your chest is opened up. Push your pelvis slightly forward, although this will be more difficult in this position. Hold your gaze parallel to the floor. (Repeat by swapping your feet over.)

Lotus Pose

Once you are comfortable being seated in the easy pose, then you can work towards the lotus position. It can be very challenging to achieve the lotus position, and so you must be patient as progress may be slow and gradual. Again, different people find that different things make achieving this position difficult. For example, some people may feel it is their ankles and knees that are holding them back. Others may feel that it is their hips. This is a very satisfying position to achieve and is well worth persevering with.

You should start from the easy pose and then place one of your feet onto the thigh. This is known as the half lotus position. You will need to become comfortable with this position before you can attempt the full lotus. When in the half lotus position, work towards bringing the raised foot as close to your hip as possible, high up onto your thigh. Also, try to turn the foot such that the sole faces upwards. Once you can comfortably accomplish this on both sides, then it is time to attempt the full lotus position.

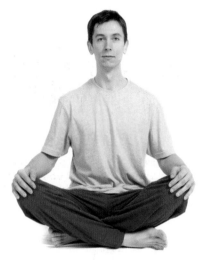

Step 1. Start in the easy pose.

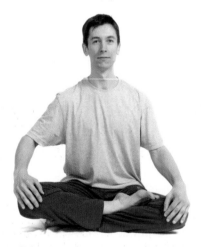

Step 2. Bring one foot to rest up onto your opposite thigh. Bring your foot in as close to your hip as possible and aim to keep both of your knees low. This position is known as the half lotus pose. Rest your hands lightly on your knees and keep your upper body relaxed. (Repeat by swapping your feet over.)

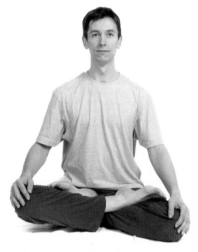

Step 3. Bring your other foot to rest onto the other thigh. Again, bring your foot in as close to your hip as possible and aim to keep both of your knees low. The soles of the feet should point upwards. Rest your hands lightly on your knees and keep your upper body relaxed. Keep your back straight and your shoulders down and pushed back slightly so that your chest is opened up. Push your pelvis slightly forward, although this will be more difficult in this position. Hold your gaze parallel to the floor. (Repeat by swapping your feet over.) In yoga, this is considered a beginner's position. However, in the West this pose is considered advanced and can take many years to master.

When you start working on the full lotus, you may find that initially you can bring both feet on top only with them crossing at the ankles. With practice, you should gradually be able to work both feet closer and closer towards the hips.

Sitting Hip Adductors Stretch

Another way to sit is with the soles of the feet pushed together. Again, some students find this a very comfortable way to sit and others find it very difficult. This exercise will help you to open up the hips and work on the knee and ankle joints. If you are working towards being able to do the side splits, then this exercise will help. With this exercise, you can stop at either step two or step three depending on where you are comfortable. When pushing on the knees in step three, you must make this action gentle. Do not bounce the knees. Let them relax into the position and allow them to drop down naturally as far as they can by releasing any tension you are holding in the legs.

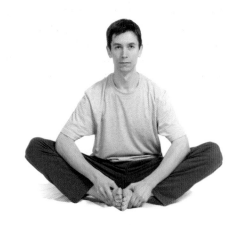

Step 2. Bring the soles of your feet together and hold with your hands. Pull your feet in as close to your body as possible. This will help you to open up your hips.

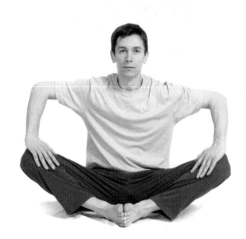

Step 3. Move your hands to your knees and gently use them to help move the knees closer to the ground. Keep your back straight and your shoulders down and pushed back slightly so that your chest is opened up. Push your pelvis slightly forward, although this will be more difficult in this position. Hold your gaze parallel to the floor.

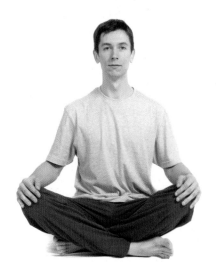

Step 1. Start in the easy pose.

Neck Exercises

Some of the following exercises may well seem simple, but it is not uncommon to lose the ability to do some of these moves as you get older. These exercises are a great way to start any training session as they are simple and relaxing. They can help you to bring your mind into the training and to leave other thoughts behind. You should feel a stretch in the sternocleidomastoid and the trapezius muscles in particular through these exercises. While doing these neck exercises, remember to:

- Keep your back upright and straight
- Rest your hands lightly on your knees or in front of you, as appropriate. Do not rest them behind you
- Keep your shoulders relaxed and down
- Do not force yourself into going too far on these exercises

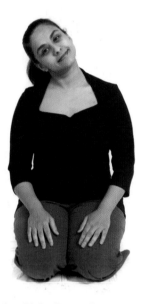

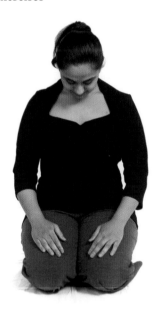

Head to the Side Stretch

Look straight ahead and then gently rest your head to one side, bringing your ear as close to your shoulder as possible. Keep your back straight and your shoulders down and pushed back slightly so that your chest is opened up. Push your pelvis slightly forward. Hold your gaze parallel to the floor. The stretch should be felt on the opposite side of your neck, in the trapezius and the sternocleidomastoid. Keep your breathing deep and let your muscles relax in the position. (Repeat on the other side.)

Head Forward Stretch

Look straight ahead and then gently rest your head forward. Keep your back straight and your shoulders down and pushed back slightly so that your chest is opened up. Push your pelvis slightly forward. Keep your shoulders relaxed and your breathing slow and deep. Bring your chin as close to your chest as possible and keep your gaze on your lap.

These simple neck exercises can be performed using any of the sitting positions described in the previous section, although they are shown here using a variant of the hero pose. You should pick whichever sitting position you are comfortable in or are working to develop and use these neck exercises to help you to work the muscles in the legs. Remember to repeat all of these exercises on both sides or in each direction as appropriate.

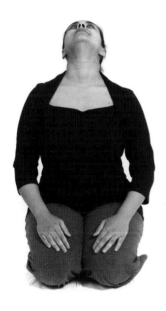

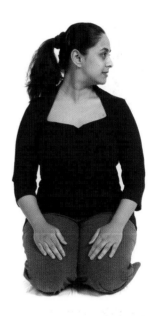

Head Back Stretch

Look straight ahead and then gently rest your head back. Keep your back straight and your shoulders down and pushed back slightly so that your chest is opened up. Push your pelvis slightly forward. Keep your shoulders relaxed and your breathing slow and deep. If you can, your eyes should look directly above you or even slightly behind you.

Head Rotation

Look straight ahead and then turn your head to look round to one side. Keep turning your head as far as you can. Keep your back straight and your shoulders down and pushed back slightly so that your chest is opened up. Push your pelvis slightly forward. Hold your gaze parallel to the floor. Keep your shoulders relaxed and your breathing slow and deep. (Repeat by rotating in the other direction.)

Wrist Exercises

These simple wrist exercises can be performed using any of the sitting positions described in the previous section, although they are shown here using a variant of the hero pose. They will help you to work your wrist joint and should feel refreshing. They are useful for people who use their hands a lot, for example writing, typing or driving.

While you may find that these are simple to do, some people find that they are quite stiff in the wrists, or have become so over time without realizing it. You should pick whichever sitting position you are comfortable in or are working to develop and use these wrist exercises to help you to work the muscles in the legs. When doing these exercises, it is important to keep the arms straight, the back upright and the shoulders down and relaxed. Remember to perform these exercises on each hand.

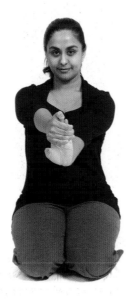

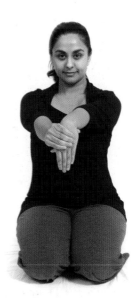

Wrist Flexor
Start with your palm facing away from you and your arm straight. Hold your palm and fingers, with your other hand, and slowly pull towards you. Keep your back straight and your shoulders down and pushed back slightly so that your chest is opened up. Push your pelvis slightly forward. Hold your gaze parallel to the floor. Keep your shoulders relaxed and your breathing slow and deep. (Repeat with your other hand.)

Wrist Extensor
Start with your palm facing towards you, then turn at your wrist so that your fingers point downwards. Hold the back of your hand, with your other hand, and gently pull towards you. Keep your back straight and your shoulders down and pushed back slightly so that your chest is opened up. Push your pelvis slightly forward. Hold your gaze parallel to the floor. Keep your shoulders relaxed and your breathing slow and deep. (Repeat with your other hand.)

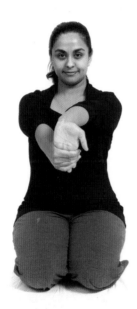 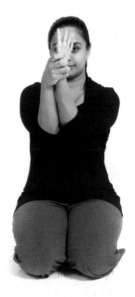

Wrist and Forearm Flexor

Start with the palm facing away from you, and then slowly rotate your hand around the outside so that your fingers point downwards. Hold your palm and fingers, with your other hand, and slowly pull towards you. Keep your back straight and your shoulders down and pushed back slightly so that your chest is opened up. Push your pelvis slightly forward. Hold your gaze parallel to the floor. Keep your shoulders relaxed and your breathing slow and deep. (Repeat with your other hand.)

Wrist Rotation

Starting with your palm facing towards you, hold the back of your hand, with your other hand, and slowly rotate your hand so that your thumb turns away from you. Keep your back straight and your shoulders down and pushed back slightly so that your chest is opened up. Push your pelvis slightly forward. Hold your gaze parallel to the floor. Keep your shoulders relaxed and your breathing slow and deep. (Repeat with your other hand.)

Arm Exercises

There are many muscles in the arm and this variety of exercises helps to develop flexibility in these areas. These arm exercises are more challenging than the wrist exercises, and they work the joints as well as the muscles. Again, it is important not to push yourself too far with these exercises. Stop at the step in the sequence before you feel any pain. Don't be fooled into thinking that these exercises are easy just because they look that way! You should pick whichever sitting position you are comfortable in or are working to develop and use these arm exercises to help you to work the muscles in the legs.

Forearm Rotation

This exercise works the muscles in the forearm and also the wrist joints. Many students don't make it all the way through the full sequence to step five. You should stop at whichever step you feel comfortable and slowly progress to the other steps as your body develops. The forearm rotation action is regularly used in sports like badminton and the martial arts. This exercise is also useful for when your arms and wrists feel tired. They can give quite a relieving stretch. You should practise this exercise on both sides.

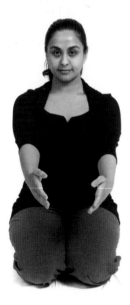

Step 1. Hold both arms out in front of you. Keep your back straight and your shoulders down and pushed back slightly so that your chest is opened up. Push your pelvis slightly forward. Hold your gaze parallel to the floor. Keep your shoulders relaxed and your breathing slow and deep.

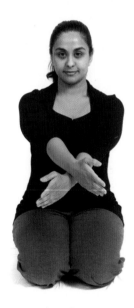

Step 2. Cross your hands over.

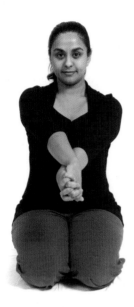

Step 3. Clasp both hands together.

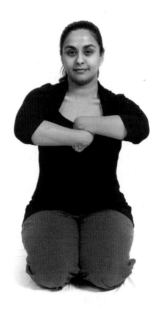

Step 4. Pull your hands in towards your body.

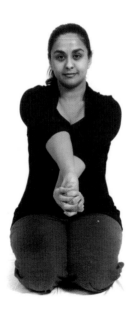

Step 5. Rotate through and try to straighten both of your arms.

Forearms Entwined

This exercise often forms part of full yoga poses. It can be incorporated, for example, into the tree pose (see Chapter 6). However, it can also be practised in isolation. This exercise predominantly works the upper arm and the wrist. Again, starting at step one, continue as far as you can comfortably go and then stop and hold this position. You can then use the later steps to give you more of a challenge as you develop. This position forms part of a number of yoga poses and can be incorporated into many balancing poses shown later in this book. This exercise should be completed on both sides.

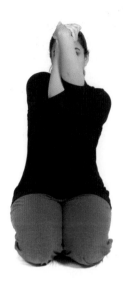

Step 2. Clasp both hands together, ensuring that there is no gap between your hands.

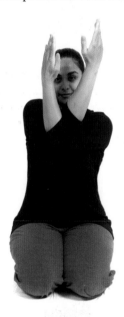

Step 1. Start by placing one elbow inside the other and bring the arm closer to you around the front of your other arm. Keep your back straight and your shoulders down and pushed back slightly so that your chest is opened up. Push your pelvis slightly forward. Hold your gaze parallel to the floor. Keep your shoulders relaxed and your breathing slow and deep.

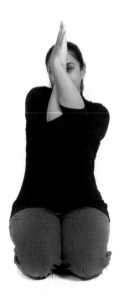

Step 3. Bring your palms together, again with no gap between your hands.

Arm Rotation

This exercise works muscles in the whole arm and also the shoulder joint. Most students find that they cannot go very far back. Many children on the other hand tend to find this exercise very easy. Once you reach your optimum position, hold for a short time before slowly bringing the arms around again in front of you. It is important not to let the arms fall below shoulder height throughout this exercise. Try to keep your back upright at all times.

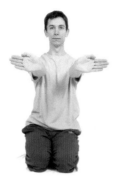

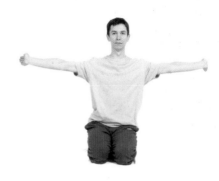

Step 1. Start with your arms out in front and your hands facing outwards. Your arms must be level with your shoulders and remember to keep your shoulders relaxed. Keep your back straight and your shoulders down and pushed back slightly so that your chest is opened up. Push your pelvis slightly forward. Hold your gaze parallel to the floor. Keep your breathing slow and deep.

Step 2. Slowly rotate your arms around behind you, while ensuring that your arms do not drop from shoulder level. If they start to drop, then come back a little bit and hold there.

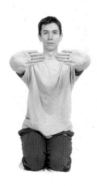

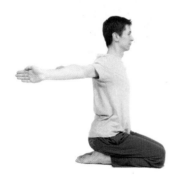

Step 3. If you can, keep going around until your arms are behind you, but still level with your shoulders.

Variant: Start from step one with your palms facing in the other direction and then work your way through steps two and three. Keep your back straight and your shoulders down and pushed back slightly so that your chest is opened up. Push your pelvis slightly forward. Hold your gaze parallel to the floor. Keep your breathing slow and deep.

Arm Lifts

This exercise works the muscles in the arms, shoulders and back. It is a very satisfying stretching position. It is useful when you have been doing poses that compress the upper body. It is also useful in helping you to work towards increasing the range of motion in your arms.

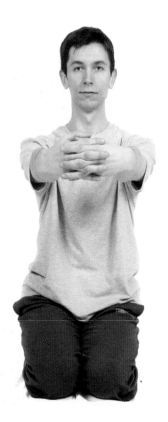

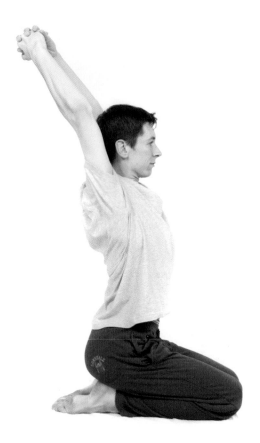

Step 1. Hold your arms out at shoulder height in front of you and interlock your fingers. Keep the elbows locked. Keep your back straight and your shoulders down and pushed back slightly so that your chest is opened up. Push your pelvis slightly forward. Hold your gaze parallel to the floor. Keep your breathing slow and deep.

Step 2. Slowly lift your arms, keeping them straight, and then push them back as far behind you as you can while keeping your arms straight.

This same exercise can be repeated, but this time starting with the arms behind you and then lift them up. This works on your shoulders in the opposite direction and is a little more difficult than the previous exercise. Again, it is a useful exercise to do after performing compressive poses and also for improving your range of motion.

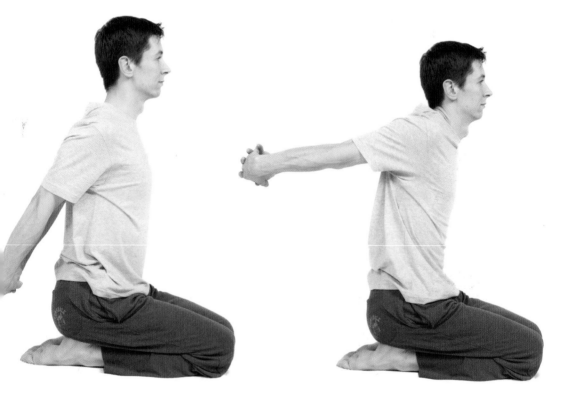

Step 1. Hold your arms out behind you and interlock your fingers. Keep the elbows locked. Keep your back straight and your shoulders down and pushed back slightly so that your chest is opened up. Push your pelvis slightly forward. Hold your gaze parallel to the floor. Keep your breathing slow and deep.

Step 2. Slowly lift your arms, keeping them straight, and then push them up as far as you can while keeping your arms straight.

Palms Together Behind Your Back

This exercise often forms part of full yoga poses and can easily be incorporated into many stretches that predominantly use the legs. It can also be practised in isolation. It works the arms, wrists and shoulders. Remember to keep your back upright and your shoulders relaxed. If you cannot bring your hands together completely, then just stop at step one and hold until you can progress further.

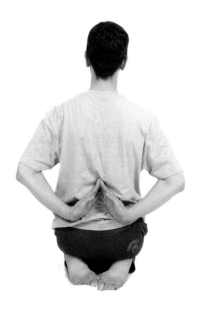

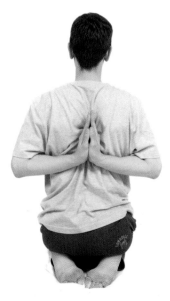

Step 1. Bring your fingers together behind your back. Keep your back straight and your shoulders down and pushed back slightly so that your chest is opened up. Push your pelvis slightly forward. Hold your gaze parallel to the floor. Keep your breathing slow and deep.

Step 2. Push your palms together so that they are flush against each other and move them up the middle of your back as far as you can without your hands coming apart.

Hands Together Behind Your Back

With practice, this exercise should enable you to reach every point on your back. It works the shoulders and upper arms. Remember to keep your back upright throughout and do not let your arms rest or push against the back of your neck or head in any of these exercises. It gives a good stretch across the back, neck and shoulders and should feel energizing.

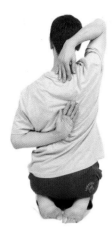 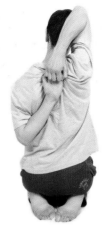

Step 1. Keep your back straight and your shoulders down and pushed back slightly so that your chest is opened up. Push your pelvis slightly forward. Hold your gaze parallel to the floor. Keep your breathing slow and deep. Place both of your hands along the middle of your back.

Step 2. Clasp your hands together in the middle of your back. (Repeat with your other arm on top.) If you can, then reach further and clasp the wrists.

If you find that it is not possible for you to bring your hands together, then you could practise the following two exercises, which will help you to build up the necessary muscles in order to achieve this exercise.

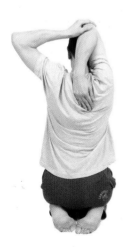 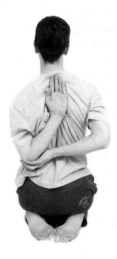

Variant 1: Push your elbow down along your spine. (Repeat with your other arm on top.)

Variant 2: Push your elbow up along your spine. (Repeat with your other arm below.)

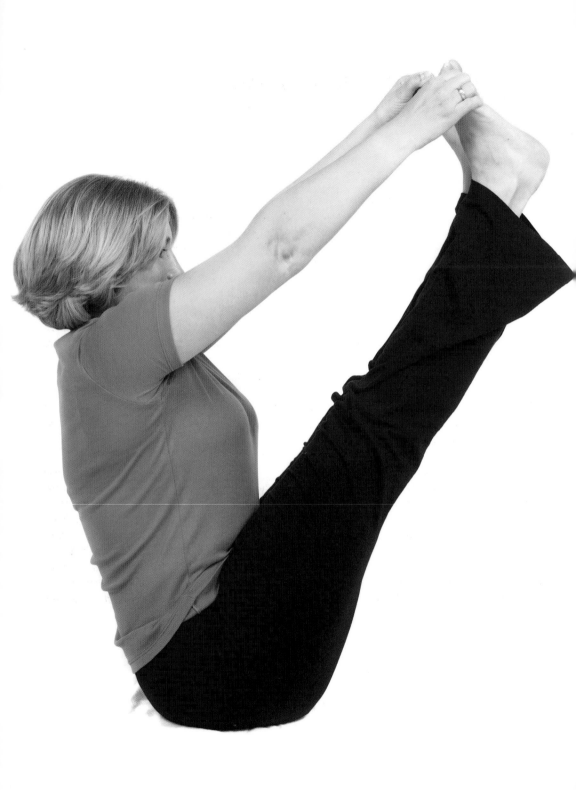

5   Seated Exercises

The seated exercises presented below are a natural follow-up to the preparation exercises (see Chapter 4). The exercises range in level of difficulty, starting off with easier exercises and moving on to more challenging poses. Despite being in a seated position, these exercises will enable you to work the whole body. They are particularly good for working on the hamstrings, the hip adductors and the back. Each of the poses is shown with step by step instructions. In general, the level of difficulty increases as you progress through the steps for each pose. The best way to practise is to start at the beginning and slowly work through the steps, stopping at the step where you can feel your muscles working effectively and being challenged at an appropriate level. It is better not to move on to later steps until you are comfortable with the earlier ones. Using this step by step approach will also give you an indication of your progress. These exercises form part of the fundamental set presented in this book that will help you towards achieving the more challenging poses presented in later chapters.

Simple feet exercises are presented as a way of working the muscles in both the front and back of the legs through a PNF approach. The poste-rior pose, a seated forward bend, is then presented in various forms, with both legs together and then variations with one leg tucked in. These seated forward bend variations are excellent for working the entire posterior of the body, and hence the name. Different variants will work different parts of the legs and back and so you should try to be aware of which muscles receive the benefit from which exercise. These exercises will also work your ankles, knees and hips. All of these forward bend exercises start using the basic staff pose position. Next exercises using the angle pose as the starting position are presented. These are excellent for working the hip adductors. The final two poses in this chapter, the lifted staff pose and the lifted angle pose, both require core strength as well as good balance.

The overall objective of the exercises in this chapter is to form a fundamental set of exercises that will help you to work on improving your overall flexibility and use of joints. They also form a core set of exercises for those wishing to achieve both the front and side splits. The quadriceps will also need to be developed in order to achieve the front splits and the exercises focusing on this muscle that are presented in later chapters.

Feet Exercises

This sequence of exercises uses PNF stretching and engages the muscles in the front and in the back of your legs through simply flexing and pointing the feet. This exercise does not require using the upper body, so keep it relaxed and just focus on the legs doing the work. This exercise is a good way to start using the muscles that will be required for the remaining poses in this chapter. It starts off in the staff pose and gets your body in position, ready for later exercises. You should proceed slowly and gently from one step to the next, giving your legs time to settle into the position before moving on. The four steps of this exercise form a sequence that can be repeated as required.

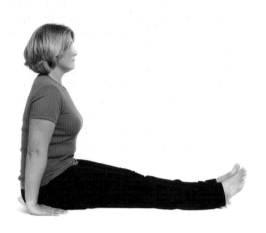

Step 1. Start in the staff pose. Place your legs a hip-width apart.

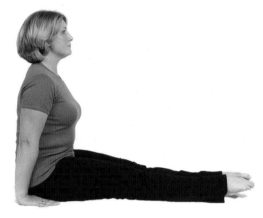

Step 2. Point your feet.

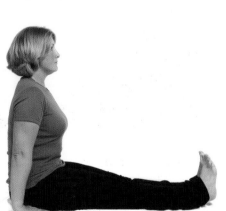

Step 3. Rest your feet in a natural position and then pull your feet back, lifting your heels off the ground.

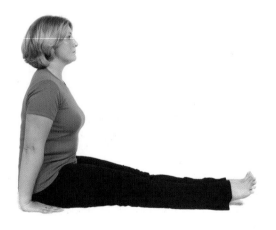

Step 4. Rest your feet in a natural position and then point your feet and pull just your toes back, letting them spread out.

Posterior Pose

This is the seated version of the forward bend, where you are aiming to reach your toes and, if you can, bend even further than that. This pose is called the posterior pose because it stretches the muscles all along the back of the body, all the way from the feet to the back of the head. The bending must be done from your hips and not from the middle of your back or your neck. If you find that you are using your neck, make sure that you look towards your feet instead of looking at your knees and this will help you to reduce the strain on your neck. Aim to get your chin to your knees rather than your nose. It should also help to reduce the risk of bending forward using your back.

The exercise starts with the staff pose and works the hands gradually forward, increasing the stretch in the back and the legs as you go. Each step represents an increasing level of difficulty. Work your way through the steps and stop where you feel you have reached a comfortable stretch. You can use these steps to give an indication of your flexibility for this particular exercise. Each step will also help you to map your progress over time. Your eventual aim should be to reach step four and rest your head down and feel comfortable in this position, reaching your heels with absolute ease and breathing without any feeling of constriction.

Step two, where you cross your hands over and hold your shins in order to help control the amount of stretch, is a good place to stop if you cannot reach your heels. Slowly increasing how much you bend at the elbow in this step will increase the stretch.

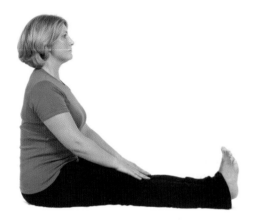

Step 1. Start in the staff pose and your heels pulled off the ground. Rest your hands on your knees and look straight ahead.

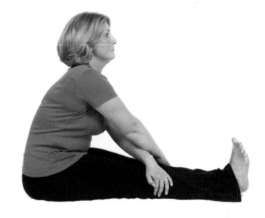

Step 2. Cross your hands over and hold your shins. Then bend your elbows in order to increase and control the stretch. Try to bend forward from the pelvic region rather than from the upper back. This should become easier with practice.

71

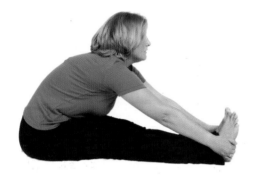

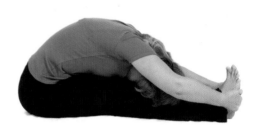

Step 3. Reach forward and cup your heels and continue to look straight ahead.

Step 4. Reach further forward and interlock your fingers around your heels and rest your head on your legs. Extend through the centre of your back and also your shoulders. Do not use your neck to pull you down.

Head to Knee Pose

This literally named pose brings the head down to rest on the knee. The exercises in this section are excellent for developing the back of the legs and the back. This is the starting position for a number of variants that can form a nice sequence. The bending must be done from your hips and not from the middle of your back or your neck. If you find that you are using your neck, make sure that you look towards your feet instead of looking at your knees and this will help to reduce the strain on your neck. It should also help to reduce the risk of bending forward using your back.

The exercise starts with the staff pose and works your hands gradually forward, increasing the stretch in your back and your legs as you go. Each step represents an increasing level of difficulty. Work your way through the steps and stop where you feel you have reached a comfortable stretch. You can use these steps to give an indication of your flexibility for this particular exercise. Each step will also help you to map your progress over time. You will want eventually to be able to reach step four and rest your head down and feel comfortable in this position, reaching your heels with absolute ease and breathing without any feeling of constriction. The two variants shown are of increasing difficulty.

Step three, where you cross your hands over and hold your shins in order to help control the amount of stretch, is a good place to stop if you cannot reach your heels. Slowly increasing how much you bend at the elbow in this step will increase the stretch.

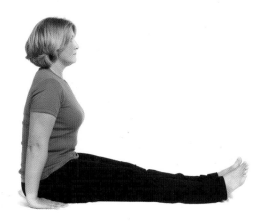

Step 1. Start in the staff pose.

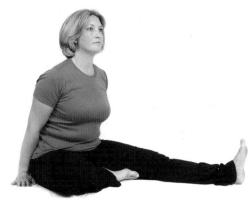

Step 2. Tuck one leg in so that your knee points out at 90 degrees. Ensure that your back is still straight by tilting your pelvis forward and pulling back your shoulders slightly to open up your chest.

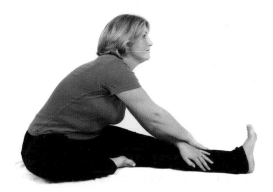

Step 3. Reach forward towards your foot, cross your arms over and rest your hands on your shins. Then bend your elbows in order to increase and control the stretch. Try to bend forward from the pelvic region rather than from your upper back or neck. This will become easier with practice. Keep your gaze parallel to the ground.

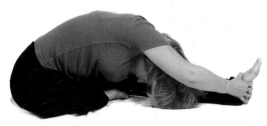

Step 4. Reach further forward and hold the heel of the outstretched leg in your hands and rest your head down. Extend through the centre of your back and also your shoulders. Do not use your neck to pull you down.

Variant 1: Using your Arms to Push Further Forward

This variation changes the stretch so that you are no longer only working the muscles on the posterior of the body. It also engages muscles on the inside of the leg. It uses the arms to push the upper body forward, rather than giving the feeling of pulling down as in the original version. It should give an increase in the stretch in your arms and shoulders as well.

Variant 2: Resting in the Centre

This variation also changes the stretch so that you are no longer working only the muscles on the posterior of the body. It also engages muscles on the inside of the leg. Resting your body between the legs will increase the stretch on the inside leg. Let your upper body and the muscles in your legs relax into the stretch. With training you should be able to push further and further forward with your hands.

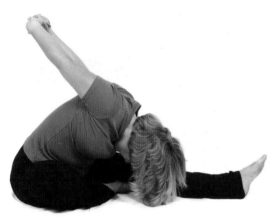

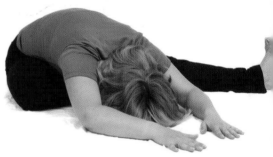

Interlock your fingers behind your back and then slowly straighten the arms. Lean forward towards the ground between your legs using your upper body. Try to bend forward from the pelvic region rather than from your upper back or neck. You should feel an intense stretch in the shoulders with this exercise.

Rest your palms on the ground between your legs. Then lean forwards and rest your forearms and your head on the ground. Try to bend forward from the pelvic region rather than from your upper back or neck. In addition to the stretch in the back of your outstretched leg, you should also feel a stretch on the inside of the outstretched leg. This combination of stretching the back and the inside of the leg at the same time can make this exercise feel quite difficult.

Revolved Head to Knee Pose

This pose changes the focus of the head to knee pose from just being on the posterior of the body to also working the side of the upper body. The final step leaves you in a comfortable and closed pose. This pose is similar to the seated gate pose (see below), except that the leg is tucked in on the inside. Each step represents an increasing level of difficulty and so you should work your way through and stop at the appropriate level.

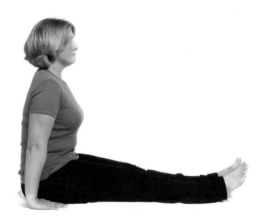

Step 1. Start in staff pose.

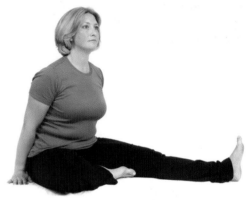

Step 2. Tuck one leg in so that your knee points out at 90 degrees. Ensure that your back is still straight by tilting your pelvis forward and pulling back your shoulders slightly to open up your chest.

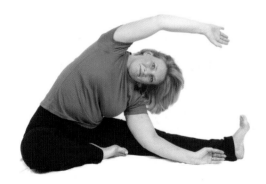

Step 3. Turn your body from your lower abdomen to bring the side of your upper body in line with your outstretched leg. Hold you arms up above your head and lean towards your leg. Try to bend along the side from the pelvic region rather than from your upper back or neck. You should feel a stretch in the side of your upper body.

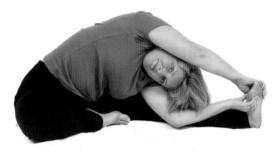

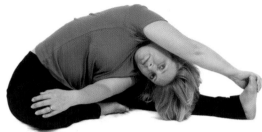

Step 4. Continue to lean forwards and hold your foot with both hands. Try to bring your elbow to rest on the ground and your shoulder to rest on your knee. This move should intensify the stretch in the side of your upper body, as well as increasing the stretch in your outstretched leg. This is the revolved head to knee pose.

Step 5. Reach towards your knee with your opposite hand and hold. This move adds an upper body twist to the position. This closes up the pose and you should feel comfortable and refreshed once it has been mastered.

Head to Knee Pose II

This is a version of the original head to knee pose. Instead of tucking the leg in on the inside, it is tucked in on the outside. It is generally more difficult than the version with the leg tucked in. This position of the legs is also known as the hurdle stretch. The same variants as suggested for the head to knee pose can be performed with this altered leg position. The hip adductors will receive a greater stretch with the leg tucked in on the outside. The two variants shown are of increasing difficulty.

Step three, where you cross your hands over and hold your shins in order to help control the amount of stretch, is a good place to stop if you cannot reach your heels. Slowly increasing how much you bend at the elbow in this step will increase the stretch.

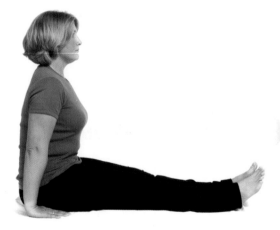

Step 1. Start in the staff pose.

76

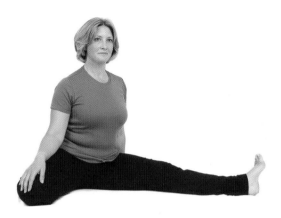

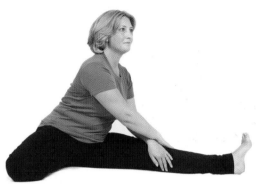

Step 2. Tuck one leg outwards so that your knee points out at 90 degrees. Ensure that your back is still straight by tilting your pelvis forward and pulling back your shoulders slightly to open up your chest.

Step 3. Reach forward towards your foot, cross your arms over and rest your hands on your shins. Then bend your elbows to help control the amount of stretch. Try to bend forward from the pelvic region rather than from your upper back or neck. This will become easier with practice. Keep your gaze parallel to the ground.

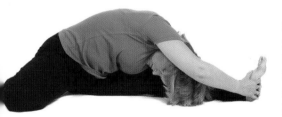

Step 4. Reach further forward and hold the heel of the outstretched leg in your hands and rest your head down. Extend through the centre of your back and also your shoulders. Do not use your neck to pull you down.

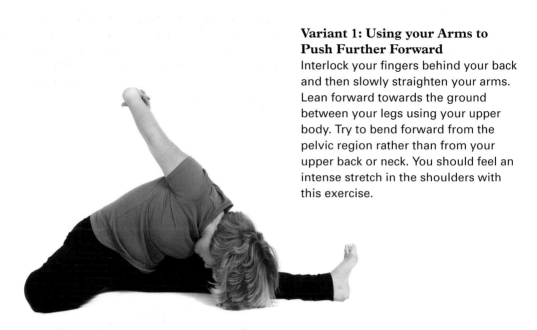

Variant 1: Using your Arms to Push Further Forward

Interlock your fingers behind your back and then slowly straighten your arms. Lean forward towards the ground between your legs using your upper body. Try to bend forward from the pelvic region rather than from your upper back or neck. You should feel an intense stretch in the shoulders with this exercise.

Variant 2: Resting in the Centre

Rest your palms on the ground between your legs. Then lean forwards and rest your forearms and your head on the ground. Try to bend forward from the pelvic region rather than from your upper back or neck. In addition to the stretch in the back of your outstretched leg, you should also feel a stretch on the inside of the outstretched leg. This combination of stretching the back and the inside of the leg at the same time can make this exercise feel quite difficult.

Seated Gate Pose

This is similar to the revolved head to knee pose (see above), except that the leg is tucked in on the outside. This pose changes the focus again from just being on the posterior of the body to working the side of the upper body. The final step leaves you in a comfortable and closed pose. Each step represents an increasing level of difficulty and so you should work your way through and stop at the appropriate level.

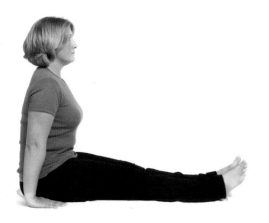

Step 1. Start in staff pose.

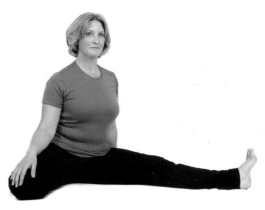

Step 2. Tuck one leg outwards so that your knee points out at 90 degrees. Ensure that your back is still straight by tilting your pelvis forward and pulling back your shoulders slightly to open up your chest.

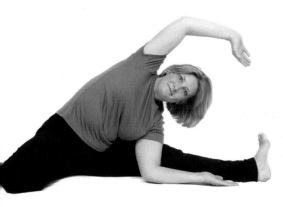

Step 3. Turn your body from your lower abdomen to bring the side of your upper body in line with the outstretched leg. Hold your arms up above your head and lean towards your leg. Try to bend along the side from the pelvic region rather than from your upper back or neck. You should feel a stretch in the side of your upper body.

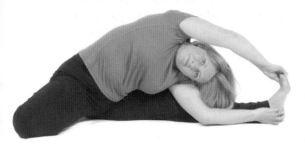 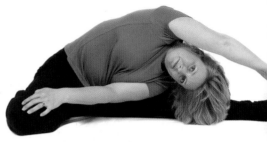

Step 4. Continue to lean forwards and hold your foot with both hands. This move should intensify the stretch in the side of your upper body, as well as increasing the stretch in your outstretched leg.

Step 5. Reach towards your knee with your opposite hand and hold. This move adds an upper body twist to the position. This closes up the pose and you should feel comfortable and refreshed once it has been mastered.

Seated Angle Pose

This pose works the inside leg and is the precursor to the more challenging yoga poses. You should work these exercises with your legs as far apart as you are comfortable and with time you should be able to see an improvement in how far you can get them apart. If you are unable to reach your feet, then you should focus your efforts on step one. Once you get to step three, you may find that you cannot push your hands very far. As you are able to separate your legs more, the easier it will become to push further forwards in step three. It is not necessary to have your legs 180 degrees apart before you are able to complete step four. These steps form the basic exercises that are required to train towards achieving the side splits.

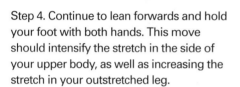
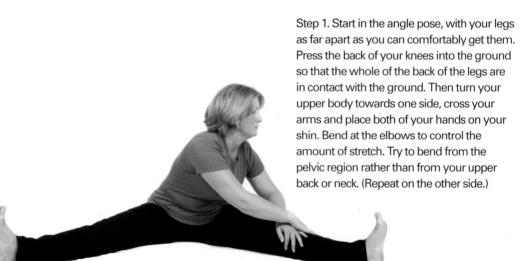

Step 1. Start in the angle pose, with your legs as far apart as you can comfortably get them. Press the back of your knees into the ground so that the whole of the back of the legs are in contact with the ground. Then turn your upper body towards one side, cross your arms and place both of your hands on your shin. Bend at the elbows to control the amount of stretch. Try to bend from the pelvic region rather than from your upper back or neck. (Repeat on the other side.)

Step 2. Reach further forward and cup the heels with both hands and bring your head down to the knee. Extend along the centre of the back and the shoulders. (Repeat on the other side.)

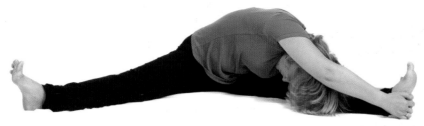

Step 3. Then rest your palms flat on the ground in front of you. Bend at the elbows and bring your forearms down to the ground and place your forehead on the ground.

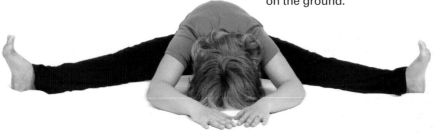

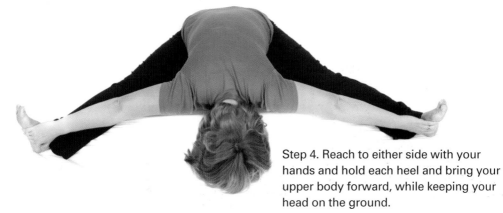

Step 4. Reach to either side with your hands and hold each heel and bring your upper body forward, while keeping your head on the ground.

Double Toe Hold Pose

This exercise is a variation of the basic staff pose. Literally named, this exercise requires you to be able to reach your toes. However, this alone will not mean that you can perform this pose. It requires precise balance and you may find that you topple over backwards for some time before you are able to balance competently on your bottom. Practising with your back against a wall may help you to master this pose.

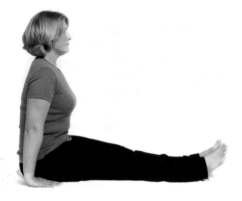

Step 1. Start in the staff pose.

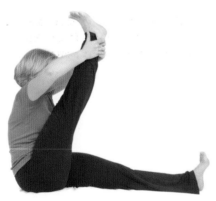

Step 2. Reach forward and hold one heel. Slowly, lift up that leg. Pause at this stage and try to balance. Keep both of your legs straight.

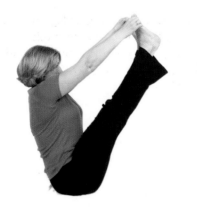

Step 3. Slowly lift up your other leg to meet your raised leg. Hold onto your toes using your hands. Focus on balancing in this position by using your core muscles and by sitting firmly on the ground. Keep your back straight.

Lifted Angle Pose

This is a variation of the double toe hold pose and it builds on the basic angle pose position. This time, instead of having the legs together and balancing, this exercise requires you to balance with the legs apart. Again, you may find that you topple over backwards for some time before you are able to balance competently on your bottom. Practising with your back against a wall may help you to master this pose.

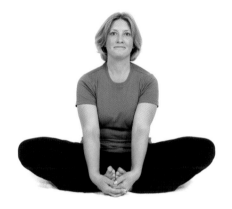

Step 1. Sit with the soles of your feet together. Keep your back straight and your shoulders down and pushed back slightly so that your chest is opened up. Push your pelvis slightly forward and bring your navel in slightly towards your spine. Hold your gaze parallel to the floor.

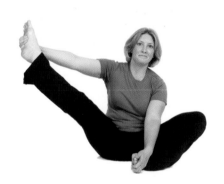

Step 2. Hold your feet with your hands and lift one leg off to the side and lock the knee. Pause at this stage and try to balance.

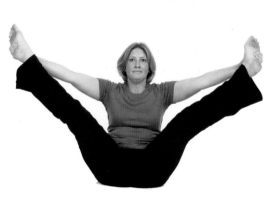

Step 3. Slowly lift your other leg and lock the knee. Focus on balancing in this position by using your core muscles and by sitting firmly on the ground. Keep your back straight.

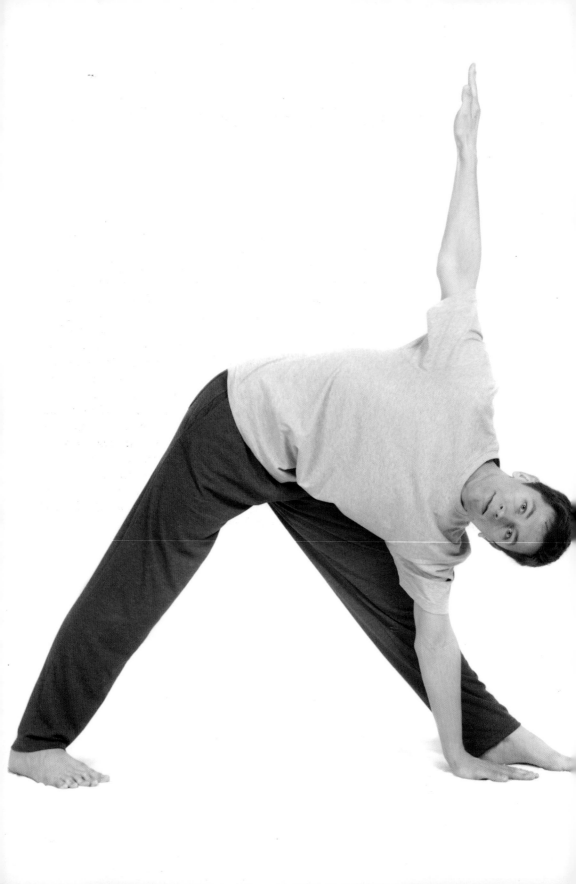

6   Standing Exercises

Standing poses are particularly good for strengthening the legs and practising your balance. Beginners may find these exercises quite difficult, however, although many of them can be modified to make them achievable for newcomers until they have developed more by using the step by step approach presented here.

We start with the forward bend pose, which is the standing version of the posterior pose (see Chapter 5). Then there are some variants of the forward bend, namely the single-legged forward bend, which works the muscles in the leading leg intensely, and then the feet-apart version of the forward bend, which works the muscles of the inside leg intensely. These exercises form a fundamental set for those working towards achieving the front splits and the side splits.

The downward-facing dog poses then add the dimension of putting weight onto the arms. These exercises will help you to strengthen the upper body as well as working the back of the legs. The staple poses of yoga training, the triangle, the warrior and their variants, are then presented. These exercises are excellent for training the body towards strengthening the legs and also improving flexibility in order to achieve the Hanuman pose, also known as the front splits. The rotated variants are excellent for working the spine.

The remaining exercises in this chapter – the tree, standing hand to toes poses, the half moon pose and the half bow pose – all require balance in addition to strength. Again, these exercises are shown using a step by step approach and also with variants, as appropriate, to enable you to modify these exercises in terms of difficulty level to suit you best.

Basic Standing Position

This is the basic starting position used for most of the standing poses presented in this chapter. It is a variation of the mountain pose, where the feet are placed together. This is a simple-looking exercise, where your focus must be on keeping the body in alignment and the upper body relaxed. It is very easy to hold tension in the shoulders and so you must actively focus your attention on keeping them down.

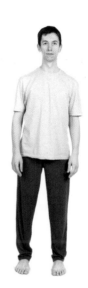

Step 1. Start in the basic standing position. Keep your back straight and your shoulders down and pushed back slightly so that your chest is opened up.

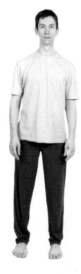

Stand with your feet a hip-width apart. Keep your back straight and your shoulders down and pushed back slightly so that your chest is opened up. Rest your arms down by your sides.

Upper Body Side Stretch

This simple exercise gives a refreshing stretch to the side of the body. You should only lean over enough to feel the stretch and not so much that you are competing to see how far you can bend over to the side. This exercise can also be used between yoga poses for loosening up the body before continuing with your practice, an excellent way to punctuate your session.

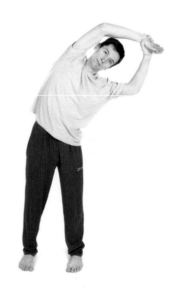

Step 2. Raise both of your arms, bringing your hands together. Then slowly lean to one side from the lower abdomen region. You should feel the stretch across the side of your body and your arm. (Repeat on the other side.)

Tree Pose

This exercise will help you to work on your balance. Also it will require you to be able to lift your foot, unsupported, to the top of your thigh. It is best to work your way through the steps and stop when you reach the stage that you feel needs some work. It may be your balance or your ability to raise your leg unsupported that holds you back from achieving this pose. Step three is the simplest form of this exercise. It is best to focus here until you are able to balance, before moving on.

Step 1. Start in the basic standing position. Keep your back straight and your shoulders down and pushed back slightly so that your chest is opened up.

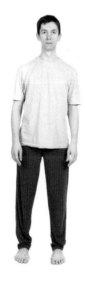

Step 2. Bring your palms together and then raise your arms above your head. Straighten the arms.

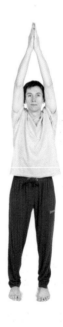

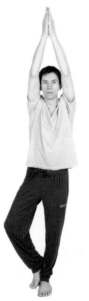

Step 3. Lift one foot up and rest it on your ankle. Ensure that your toes point downwards and that your knee points out to the side.

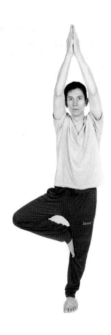

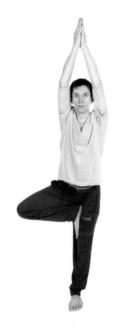

Step 4. Raise your foot and rest it on your knee. Again, ensure that your toes point downwards and that your knee points out to the side.

Step 5. Raise your foot further and rest it on the inside of your upper thigh, reaching as high as you can. Keep your gaze parallel to the ground and focus on balancing in this position.

Forward Bend Pose

This pose is the standing version of the posterior pose (see Chapter 5). It works the muscles in the back of the body intensely. In addition, this standing version requires you to balance in position. Since it also results in inverting your head, if you feel any uneasiness when performing this exercise, you must stop immediately and speak to your instructor. In general, all the contraindications given for inverted poses apply to this exercise. If you are unable to reach the ground in this exercise, then you should stop at step three and work towards lowering your upper body further before attempting the remaining steps. You can also try using blocks to give you support.

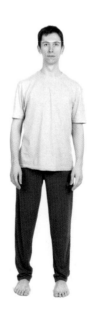

Step 1. Start in the basic standing position.

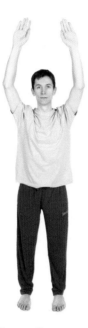

Step 2. Lift your arms straight above your head and stretch upwards, keeping your feet flat on the ground. You should feel your back and shoulders extending.

Step 3. Interlock your fingers and, keeping the knees locked, rest your upper body down. Keep the muscles in the upper body relaxed and let your weight bring you down.

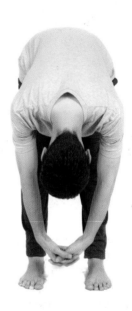

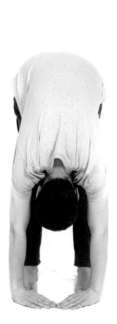

Step 4. Slowly reach further down and place your palms flat on the ground in front of you and about a hip-width apart. Bend forward from the pelvic region rather than the upper back and neck.

89

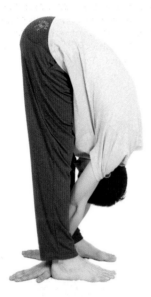

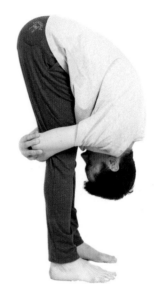

Step 5. Reach through between your feet and rest your palms on the ground behind your feet. Try to bring your wrists in contact with your heels and point the fingers backwards.

Step 6. Bring your arms behind your legs, keeping the knees locked, and bring your hands to rest on your elbows. Focus on your balance and keeping your breathing steady.

Single Leg Forward Bend Pose

This variation of the forward bend works the hamstrings in the leading leg intensely. This series of steps should be repeated on both sides. If you are unable to reach the ground, then you can interlock your fingers and just let the arms rest down in front of you. You can also try using blocks to give you support. Relax your upper body and let your weight help to bring you further down. Adding your arms to the exercise in steps three and four will enable you to also work the shoulders intensely at the same time.

This exercise also results in inverting your head, so if you feel any uneasiness when performing it you must stop immediately and speak to your instructor. In general, all the contraindications given for inverted poses apply to this exercise.

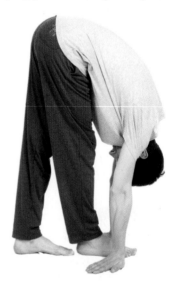

Step 1. Start with your feet heel to toe and then, keeping the knees locked, bend forward and rest your palms flat on the ground next to your leading foot. Remember to bend forward from your pelvic region and not the upper body.

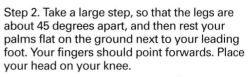

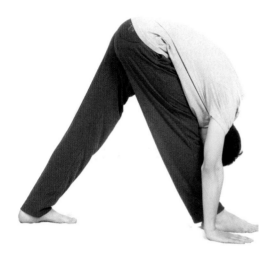

Step 2. Take a large step, so that the legs are about 45 degrees apart, and then rest your palms flat on the ground next to your leading foot. Your fingers should point forwards. Place your head on your knee.

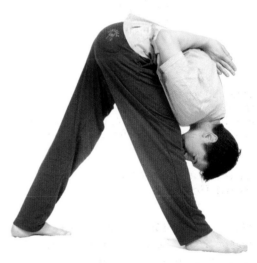

Step 3. Bring your palms together behind your back while keeping your head on your knee. Push your palms as far up the middle of your back as you can reach.

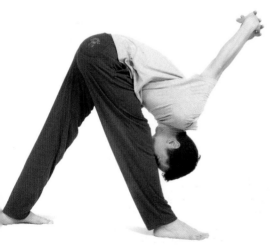

Step 4. Then, interlocking your fingers, straighten your arms and use them to push your upper body further down. You should feel an intense stretch in your shoulders and upper back.

Feet Apart Forward Bend Pose

This exercise is more difficult than the previous forward bend as it also stretches the inside leg. This is like a standing version of the angle pose from the previous chapter. Being in a standing position has the additional benefit of being able to use your body weight to help with the stretch. If you are unable to reach the ground, then you can interlock your fingers and just let the arms rest down in front of you. You can also try using blocks to give you support. Relax the upper body and let your weight help to bring you further down.

This is an excellent exercise for those interested in improving their inside leg flexibility and those looking to work towards the side splits. The key to this exercise is to keep the knees locked throughout. You should widen the distance that your feet are apart as you progress. Once you are able to reach step eight, you can focus on pushing the upper body forward to help you to push your legs wider. This exercise also results in inverting your head, so if you feel any uneasiness when performing it you must stop immediately and speak to your instructor. In general, all the contraindications given for inverted poses apply to this exercise.

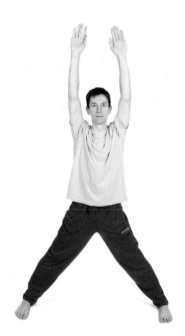

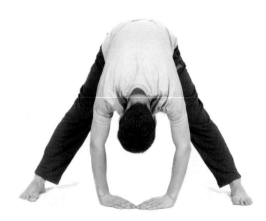

Step 1. Start with your feet apart, so that your legs are at about 90 degrees, with your back straight and your shoulders pulled slightly back to open up your chest. Your toes should point forwards. Keep your knees locked throughout this exercise. Lift and straighten your arms above your head.

Step 2. Slowly reach forward and down, bending from your pelvic region. Place your palms flat on the ground in front of you and in line with your toes.

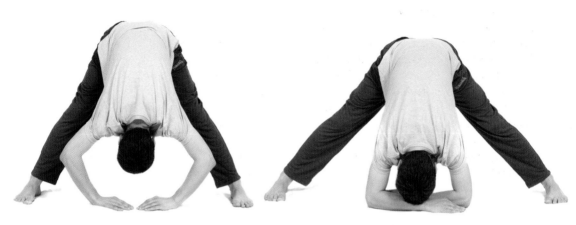

Step 3. Bend at the elbows and use the action to bring your upper body further down. Remember to bend from the pelvic region and not from the upper back.

Step 4. Push your legs to as far apart as you are comfortable, while still being able to remain standing. Place your forearms and your head on the ground. Your forearms should be just in front of your toes on the ground.

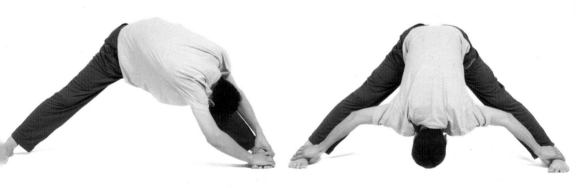

Step 5. Reach over to one side and hold your foot with both hands and rest your head on your knee. Keep your knees locked and your feet firmly on the ground with your toes pointing forwards. (Repeat on the other side.)

Step 6. Hold both of your feet and place your head down on the ground. Focus on keeping your breathing steady.

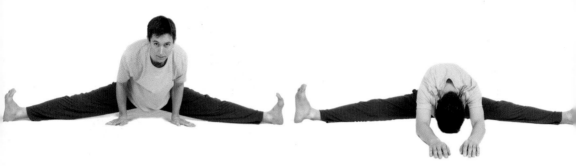

Step 7. Place your hands on the ground, near your centre and about a hip-width apart, and lift your weight up onto your heels and push wider. Support your weight on your hands and on your heels.

Step 8. Slowly sit down onto the floor, bring your upper body to rest on the ground and push your arms forward. Extend through your back and shoulders. Keep your feet pulled back so that your toes are pointing upward.

Downward-Facing Dog Pose

This exercise gives an intense stretch in the hamstrings, calves, back and shoulders. This position will also develop your arm strength, as much weight is placed on the hands. As a result, holding this position for increasing amounts of time will require much arm strength. This pose forms part of the sun salutation sequence (see Chapter 8).

This exercise results in inverting your head, so if you feel any uneasiness when performing it you must stop immediately and speak to your instructor. In general, all the contraindications given for inverted poses apply to this exercise.

If you are unable to reach the floor with your hands in order to perform this exercise, then you can try using blocks under your hands. This should enable you to continue to get into the same position and stretch your legs and back, even though your hands cannot reach the ground yet.

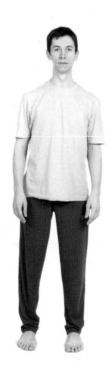

Step 1. Start in the basic standing position. Your feet should be a hip-width apart.

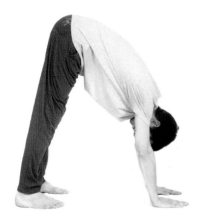

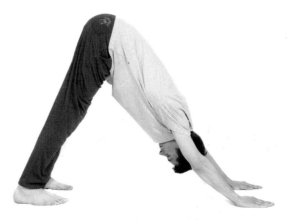

Step 2. Bend forward and place your palms on the ground while keeping your legs straight. Then work your hands forward. Point the fingers forward.

Step 3. Push back, so that your upper body is straightened and your head is in line with your arms. Your hands and feet should be firmly on the ground. Do not let your heels lift up; instead actively push the heels into the ground. This pose works the muscles in the posterior of the body.

One-Legged Downward-Facing Dog Pose

This exercise also gives an intense stretch in the hamstrings, calves, back and shoulders. This position will develop your arm strength, since much weight is placed on the hands, even more so than in the downward-facing dog pose. As a result, holding this position for increasing amounts of time will require much arm strength.

This exercise results in inverting your head, so if you feel any uneasiness when performing it you must stop immediately and speak to your instructor. In general, all the contraindications given for inverted poses apply to this exercise.

If you are unable to reach the floor with your hands in order to perform this exercise, then you can try using blocks under your hands. This should enable you to continue to get into the same position and stretch with the legs and back, even though your hands cannot reach the ground yet.

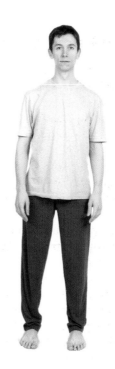

Step 1. Start in the basic standing position. Your feet should be a hip-width apart.

Step 2. Bend forward from your pelvic region and place your palms on the ground while keeping your legs straight. Then work your hands forward. Point the fingers forward.

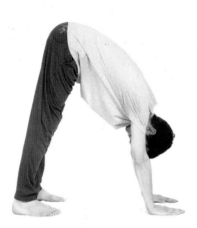

Step 3. Push back, so that your upper body is straightened and your head is in line with your arms. Your hands and feet should be firmly on the ground. Do not let your heels lift up; instead actively push the heels into the ground.

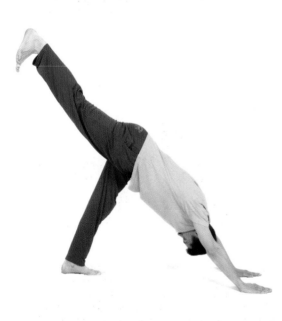

Step 4. Slowly lift one of your legs and bring it in line with your upper body. Do not move the upper body out of position. Keep both knees locked. (Repeat on the other side.)

Triangle Pose

This pose works the back of the leading leg and also develops your awareness of alignment and posture. If you are unable to reach the ground in step three, then you could attempt this exercise with the use of a block under your hand. These various steps can be joined together into a sequence of increasing difficulty. The variant shown is slightly more difficult than step three, since it requires a slight turning of the upper body in order to place the hand on the other side of the foot.

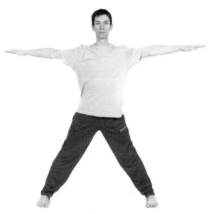

Step 1. Start with your feet about two to three shoulder-widths apart (you want to form about 90 degrees with your legs), your back straight and your shoulders relaxed. Your toes should point forwards. Raise your arms to bring them in line with your shoulders and pointing out to the side. Your palms should face down.

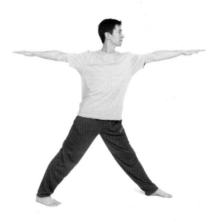

Step 2. Turn your feet to point to the side and look along your leading arm. Your leading foot should point directly forwards and your rear foot should point about 45 degrees off to the side, so that it is in a natural position. Keep both legs straight.

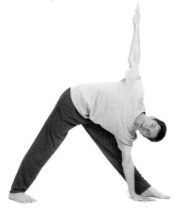

Step 3. Bend your upper body sideways and rest your palm flat on the ground with the fingers pointing forwards, alongside the inside of your leading foot. Your other arm should point vertically upwards and be in line with your supporting arm. (Repeat on the other side.)

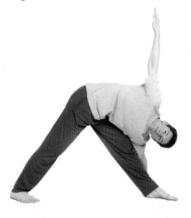

Variant: Place your palm flat on the ground with the fingers pointing forwards, alongside the outside of your leading foot. Your other arm should point vertically upwards and be in line with your supporting arm. (Repeat on the other side.)

Rotated Triangle Pose

This is the rotated form of the triangle, where the upper body is rotated so that a twist is worked into the pose. This rotated version is generally more difficult than the straightforward version of the triangle. This pose works the back of the leading leg and also develops your awareness of alignment and posture. If you are unable to reach the ground in step four, then you could attempt this exercise with the use of a block under your hand. These various steps can be joined together into a sequence of increasing difficulty. The variant shown is slightly more difficult than step four, since it requires a slight turning of the upper body in order to place the hand on the other side of the foot.

Step 1. Start with your feet about two to three shoulder-widths apart (you want to form about 90 degrees with your legs), your back straight and your shoulders relaxed. Your toes should point forwards. Raise your arms to bring them in line with your shoulders and pointing out to the side. Your palms should face down.

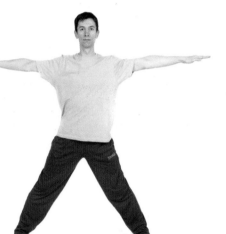

Step 2. Turn your feet to point to the side and look along your leading arm. Your leading foot should point directly forwards and your rear foot should point about 45 degrees off to the side, so that it is in a natural position. Keep both legs straight.

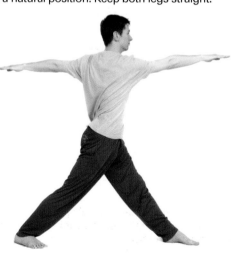

Step 3. Rotate your upper body, so that your rear arm swings around to point forward. This move adds an upper body twist.

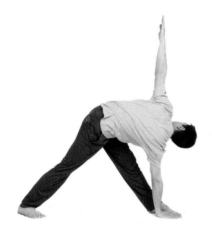

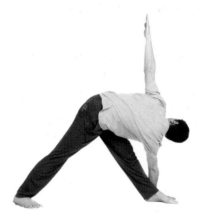

Step 4. Bend your upper body sideways and rest your palm flat on the ground with the fingers pointing forwards, alongside the inside of your leading foot. Your other arm should point vertically upwards and be in line with your supporting arm. (Repeat on the other side.)

Variant: Place your palm flat on the ground with the fingers pointing forwards, alongside the outside of your leading foot. Your other arm should point vertically upwards and be in line with your supporting arm. (Repeat on the other side.)

Warrior Poses

Warrior I Pose
This pose strengthens the legs and stretches the back and shoulders. The lower you can hold your body, the greater effort will be required in order to hold this pose. With practice, you should be able to hold this pose for increasing lengths of time.

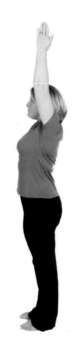

The Naming of the Warrior Pose

This pose is named after a great warrior who rose up from Lord Siva's hair. This warrior led Siva's army in order to avenge the death of Siva's wife. The three versions of the warrior pose, dedicated to this great hero, form part of the fundamentals for achieving more challenging poses.

Step 1. Start in the basic standing position. Then lift your arms straight above your head and bring your palms together.

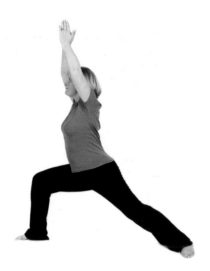

Step 2. Take one large step forward, so that the thigh of your front leg is parallel to the ground and you cannot see your toes from over your knees. Your front foot should point forwards and your rear foot should point naturally off to the side, about 45 degrees. Keep your gaze parallel to the ground. Keep your back upright. Do not lean into the pose. This is a strenuous pose and you should be aware of how your muscles are coping with this exercise.

Warrior II Pose

This is the second of the warrior poses and here the arms are held out to the side in line with the shoulders. This pose strengthens the legs and stretches the back and shoulders. The lower you can hold your body, the greater effort will be required in order to hold this pose. With practice, you should be able to hold this pose for increasing lengths of time. This pose helps you to work on your body awareness in terms of knowing when your arms are in line with your shoulders. If you are able to practice in front of a mirror, then you can use that to check your own alignment.

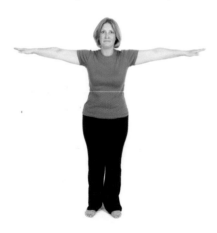

Step 1. Start in the basic standing position. Then bring your arms in line with your shoulders with the palms facing down.

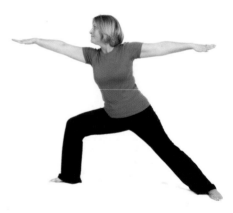

Step 2. Turn to look to one side and take a step forward. Bring the thigh of your leading leg parallel to the ground. You should not be able to see your toes over your knees. Your front foot should point forwards and your rear foot should point naturally off to the side, about 45 degrees. Keep your gaze parallel to the ground. Keep your back upright. Do not lean into the pose. This is a strenuous pose and you should be aware of how your muscles are coping with this exercise.

The four variants illustrated require placing your hand on the ground. If you are unable to reach the ground, then you could attempt these exercises with the use of a block under your hand. These have the additional benefit of working on your awareness of your alignment as well as stretching the side of the upper body.

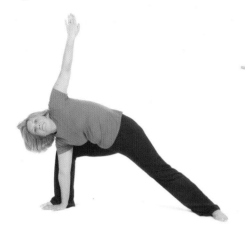

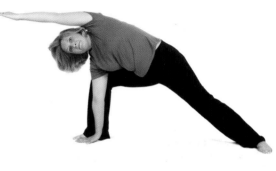

Variant 1: Rest your palm down on the ground on the inside and reach upwards with your other arm. The fingers of your supporting hand should point forwards.

Variant 2: Rest your palm down on the ground on the inside and reach in line with your upper body. This should give you an intense stretch across the side of your upper body. The fingers of your supporting hand should point forwards.

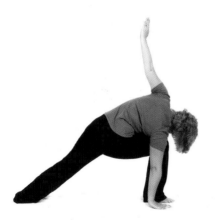

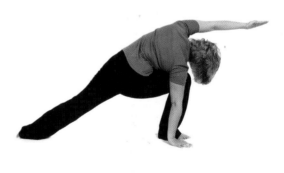

Variant 3: Rest your palm down on the ground on the outside and reach upwards with your other arm. The fingers of your supporting hand should point forwards. This exercise is more difficult due to the supporting hand being on the outside rather than the inside.

Variant 4: Rest your palm down on the ground on the outside and reach in line with your upper body. The fingers of your supporting hand should point forwards. This should give you an intense stretch across the side of your upper body. This exercise is more difficult due to the supporting hand being on the outside rather than the inside.

Rotated Warrior II Pose

These exercises are the same as the warrior II pose, except that a rotation in the upper body has been added. This makes this set of exercises slightly more difficult than those of the straightforward warrior II pose. Again, for the variant exercises, if you are unable to reach the ground, then you could attempt these exercises with the use of a block under your hand.

Step 1. Start in the basic standing position. Then bring your arms in line with your shoulders with the palms facing down.

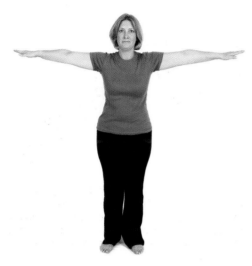

Step 2. Turn to look to one side and take a step forward. Bring the thigh of your leading leg parallel to the ground. You should not be able to see your toes over your knees. Your front foot should point forwards and your rear foot should point naturally off to the side, about 45 degrees. Keep your gaze parallel to the ground. Keep your back upright. Do not lean into the pose.

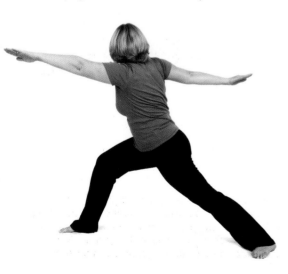

Step 3. Rotate your upper body, so that your rear arm swings around to point forward. This move adds an upper body twist.

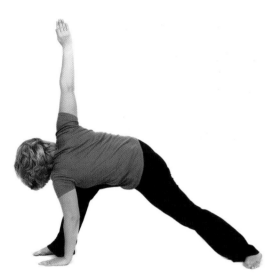

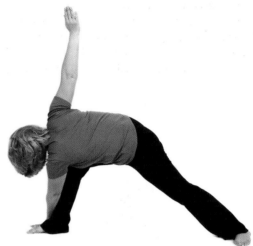

Variant 1: Rest your palm down on the ground on the inside and reach upwards with your other arm. The fingers of your supporting hand should point forwards.

Variant 2: Rest your palm down on the ground on the outside and reach upwards with your other arm. The fingers of your supporting hand should point forwards. This exercise is more difficult due to the supporting hand being on the outside rather than the inside.

Warrior III Pose

This final warrior pose requires the use of balance as well as a good understanding of body alignment. You will need to ensure that your whole body is parallel to the ground and perpendicular to your supporting leg. If you are able to practise in front of a mirror, then you can use that to check your own alignment.

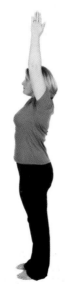

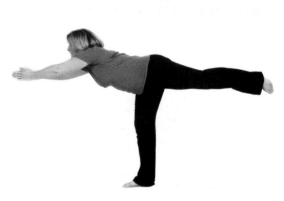

Step 1. Start in the basic standing position. Then lift your arms straight above your head and bring your palms together.

Step 2. Keeping one leg on the ground, lean forward from your middle and lift your other leg off the ground. Continue leaning until your upper body and leg are parallel to the ground. Keep your gaze parallel to the ground and balance.

Hanuman (Monkey God) Pose

This pose resembles the front splits and gives an intensive stretch to the hamstrings and the quadriceps. It should be practised on either side of the body.

The Naming of the Hanuman Pose

This pose is named after the monkey god that served Ram and Laksman. The pose is supposed to represent the leaps that the monkey would perform during its service to Ram and Laksman.

If you are new to this type of exercise, then it is best that you work on step three.

Here you are pushing the front leg forward and the rear leg backward. In the beginning, you will probably start with your back knee on the ground. With time you should be able to progress by beginning to bring your rear thigh onto the ground. It will take time to master this pose and be able to sit comfortably on the ground in it. Up to step four, you will be supporting much of your weight on your hands. When you reach step five, where you lift your hands off the ground, you will put greater pressure onto your legs and this will act in challenging your body to go lower still.

It is important not to let your body turn or drop to one side when performing this exercise, as it will give you a false sense of achievement and you will not be working the correct muscles that are needed to perform this exercise successfully.

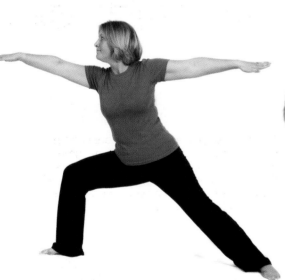

Step 1. Start in the warrior II pose.

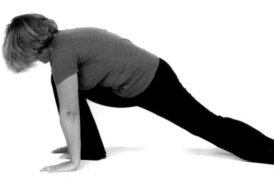

Step 2. Place your palms down on the ground near your front foot with your fingers pointing forwards.

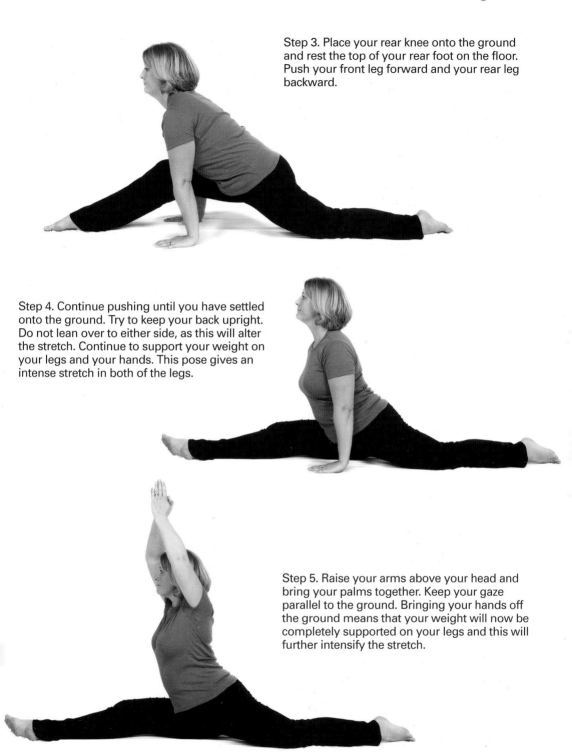

Step 3. Place your rear knee onto the ground and rest the top of your rear foot on the floor. Push your front leg forward and your rear leg backward.

Step 4. Continue pushing until you have settled onto the ground. Try to keep your back upright. Do not lean over to either side, as this will alter the stretch. Continue to support your weight on your legs and your hands. This pose gives an intense stretch in both of the legs.

Step 5. Raise your arms above your head and bring your palms together. Keep your gaze parallel to the ground. Bringing your hands off the ground means that your weight will now be completely supported on your legs and this will further intensify the stretch.

Extended Hand to Toe Pose

This literally named exercise requires both strength and balance in order to hold this position. You must keep the knee locked in this exercise. Start by lifting the leg to just your waist height and then slowly bring your foot higher, as far as your flexibility and strength allows. This exercise works the body quite intensely.

If you are unable to reach your foot while keeping the raised leg straight, then you could consider using straps to help you reach your foot. This exercise works the muscles in the back of the raised leg. Remember to practise this exercise equally on both sides.

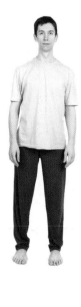

Step 1. Start in the basic standing position.

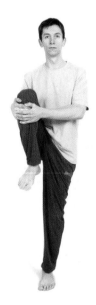

Step 2. Bring your knee as close to your chest as possible, supporting it with both hands.

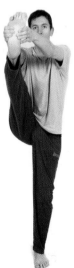

Step 3. Holding the foot, straighten your leg out in front of you. You can slightly bend the supporting leg to help you balance. Keep your gaze parallel to the ground.

Side Extended Hand to Toe

This exercise is similar to the extended hand to toe pose, except that this time you will extend your leg out to the side of your body.

This exercise requires both strength and balance and it will, in addition to the hamstrings, work the hip adductors. Remember to practise this exercise equally on both sides.

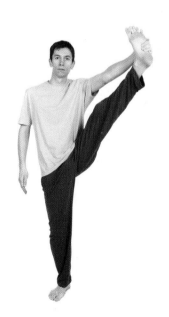

Step 1. Start in the basic standing position.

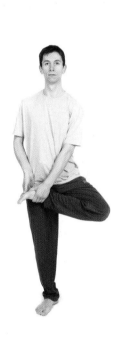

Step 2. Bring your foot as close to your hip as possible, supporting it with both hands. The sole of your foot should point upwards and your raised knee should point out to the side.

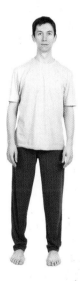

Step 3. Extend your leg out to the side while holding with one hand. Your extended leg should be straight. You can slightly bend the supporting leg to help you balance. Keep your gaze parallel to the ground.

107

Half Moon Pose

This standing pose requires you to balance on one hand and one foot. It is so named as it is believed that the pose takes the shape of a half moon. If you are unable to reach the ground with your hand, then you may wish to use a block to support you in this exercise. It is useful to perform this pose in front of a mirror in order to help you with alignment. This is particularly the case with the variant shown here, which straightens your other arm, bringing it in line with your supporting arm. Remember to practise this exercise equally on both sides.

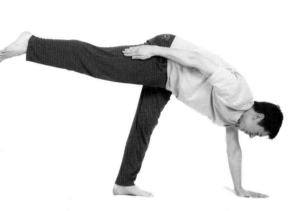

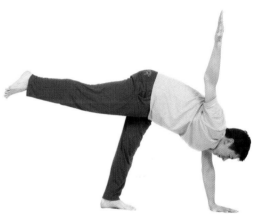

Step 1. Slowly lift one leg and bring the hand on the supporting leg side down to rest on the ground in front of you. Your supporting leg should be straight. Keep your other arm in line with your body. The raised leg should be parallel to the ground and the fingers of the supporting hand should point forwards. Once in this position, focus on your balance.

Variant: Point the other arm vertically upwards and keep it in line with your supporting arm. Your supporting leg should be straight. Once in this position, focus on your balance.

Rotated Half Moon Pose

This pose is similar to the half moon pose, except that the opposite arm to the leg is used for support on the ground. This rotation means that your back gets an additional workout from this version of the exercise. If you are unable to reach the ground with your hand, then you may wish to use a block to support you in this exercise. It is useful to perform this pose in front of a mirror in order to help you with alignment. Remember to practise this exercise equally on both sides.

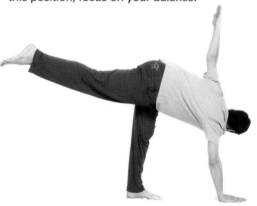

Slowly lift one leg and bring your hand, on the opposite side of your supporting leg, down to rest on the ground in front of you. Point the other arm upwards and keep it in line with the supporting arm. Your raised leg should be parallel with the ground and the fingers of your supporting hand should point forwards. Your supporting leg should be straight.

Standing Half Bow Pose

This exercise is the precursor to more advanced poses in a similar vein that require the spine to be able to bend comfortably into a concave shape. This exercise requires balance, strength and an awareness of your alignment for mastery. Do not proceed to a later step until you can complete all of the previous ones perfectly competently. Remember to practise this exercise equally on both sides.

Step 1. Bend one leg at the knee, hold the foot with both hands and bring it in close to your bottom. Keep your gaze parallel to the ground.

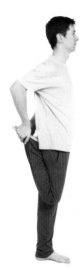

Step 2. Keeping hold of the foot with both hands, raise your leg behind you.

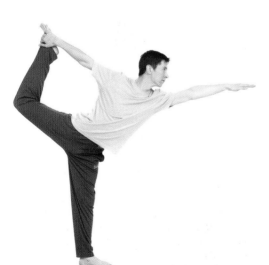

Step 3. Straighten your upper body and bring your arm on the side of your supporting leg in front of you and parallel to the ground. Raise your rear leg as high as possible and look along your leading arm.

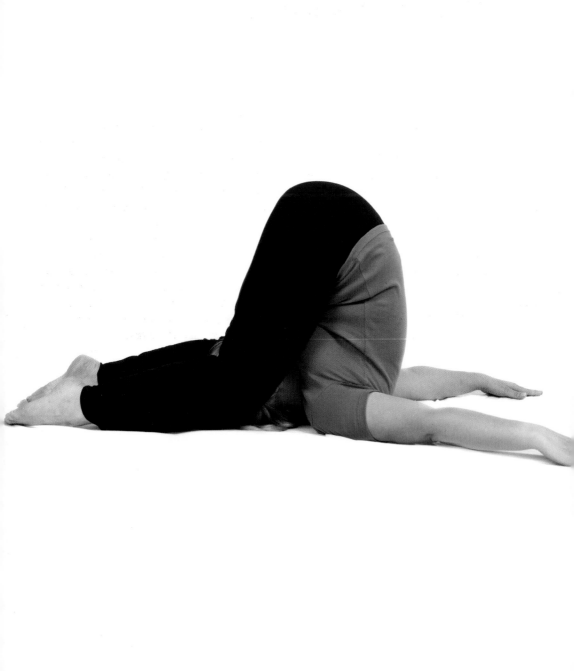

7   Supine Exercises

Poses that require you to lie on your back can be greatly relaxing. This chapter starts with the corpse pose, also known as the dead pose. This exercise, although physically simple, requires much concentration and focus in order to steady your mind. This exercise is commonly used at the end of the class in relaxation sequences. It can equally be used in between more demanding poses in order to allow the body and mind to be refreshed before progressing to more challenging poses.

The knee to chest pose is another exercise that can be used for relaxation. It has a great sense of rejuvenation about it, as the gentle twists in the body help to relieve any stress in the back. The remaining poses in this chapter are of increasing difficulty. The supine hand to toe pose and the supine angle pose both focus on working the legs, the hamstrings and the inside leg respectively.

Finally, this chapter presents the shoulder stand and a number of related exercises. These are not recommended for complete beginners. These inverted exercises in particular carry a number of contraindications that were presented in Chapter 2. Therefore, it is recommended that you ensure that you are fit to participate in these exercises. If you are unsure, you should seek professional medical advice first.

Corpse Pose

This exercise is also commonly known as the dead pose or the resting pose. Although it looks simple, it is no excuse to have a sleep! This pose is an excellent one for working on being able to steady your mind. During this exercise, you should focus on sequentially and actively relaxing the muscles throughout your body. Practise slow and deep breathing and try to free your mind of all external concerns. Many instructors use the pose to either start or end lessons. It helps to prepare the mind ready for the class and to relax you before you go back to your daily activities.

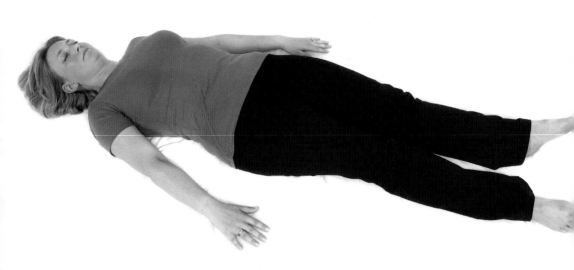

Lie on the ground with your arms resting naturally by your side and your legs comfortably apart. Try to rest your sacrum on the ground. Let your feet lie in a natural position. Focus on successively relaxing each part of your body and letting it sink into the ground.

Knees to Chest

This exercise gently works the spine. It is another great exercise for using in a relaxation sequence or for punctuating between more demanding poses. Focus on letting the muscles in your body relax during this pose and let your breathing become slow and deep. Repeat this exercise several times, taking your time to move from one side to the other.

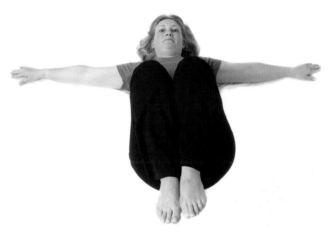

Step 1. Lie on your back, keep your feet together and bring your knees towards your chest. Place your arms straight on the ground, in line with your shoulders. Your palms should be flat on the ground.

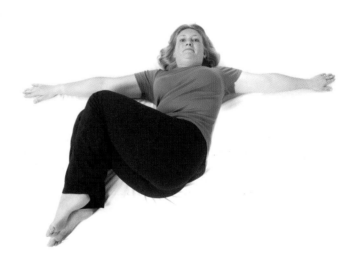

Step 2. Rest your knees onto the ground on one side, keeping your shoulders flat on the ground. This move adds a gentle twist in the back.

Supine Hand to Toe Pose

This simple-looking exercise can be quite challenging. It works the abdomen and the muscles in the legs. Perform this exercise by slowly moving into the pose, holding and then out again. You may wish to use a strap for this exercise, if you are unable to reach your feet. Remember to practise this exercise equally on both sides.

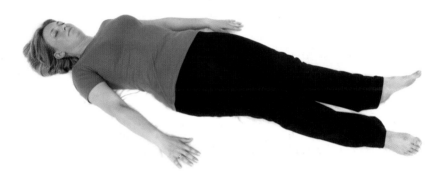

Step 1. Start in the corpse pose.

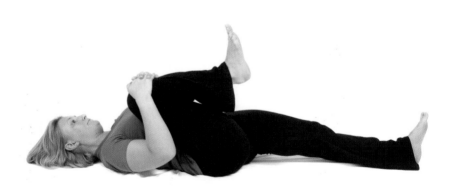

Step 2. Pull your feet back and ensure that your legs do not rotate away from the centre line. Bring one knee into your chest and hold it with your hands. Keep the other leg as straight as possible.

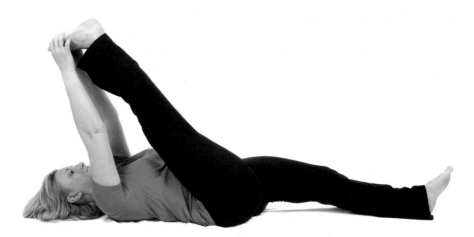

Step 3. Bring your hands to your raised foot and then straighten your leg. Pull your leg in as close to your upper body as possible. Keep the other leg firmly on the ground and as straight as possible. Do not let your body lean over to one side or the other.

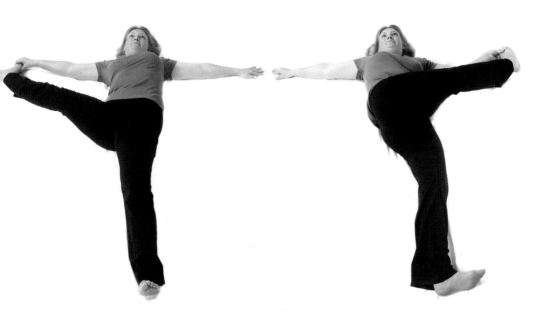

Step 4. Holding your foot with the hand on the same side as your raised leg, rest your leg on the ground, with your other arm resting on the other side, with the palm flat on the ground, in line with your shoulder.

Step 5. Holding your foot with the opposite hand, rest your leg on the ground, with your other arm resting on the other side, with the palm flat on the ground, in line with your shoulder. This move adds a gentle twist in the back.

Supine Staff Pose

This simple-looking exercise works the abdomen and the leg muscles. It has a strengthening effect the longer you hold the pose. If you are unable to hold this position, you could try aligning yourself against a wall to provide you with support.

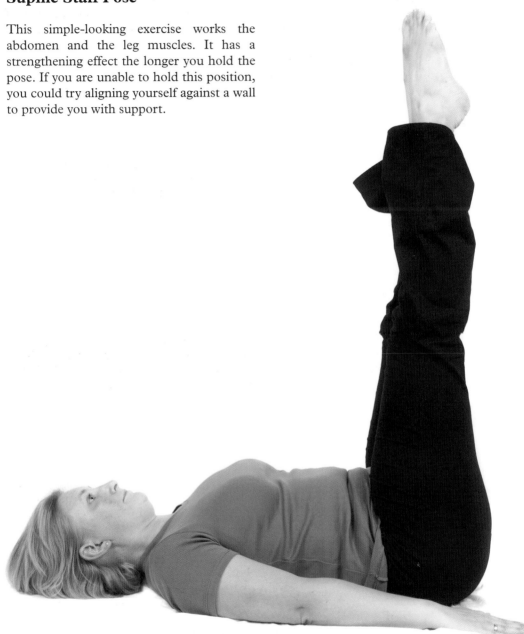

Start by lying on the ground with your arms by your side and your feet pointed. Keep your feet together. Then slowly lift your legs, so that they point upwards.

Supine Angle Pose

This exercise can also be done against a wall or without the supporting wall. It is an excellent exercise for opening the hips and working the hip adductors. As you hold this position, you may feel stress build up near the inside of the knee. Flexing the knees when coming out of this pose will help to relieve this soreness. This exercise uses your own body weight to enhance the stretch. Listen to your body to understand how long you can stay in this pose.

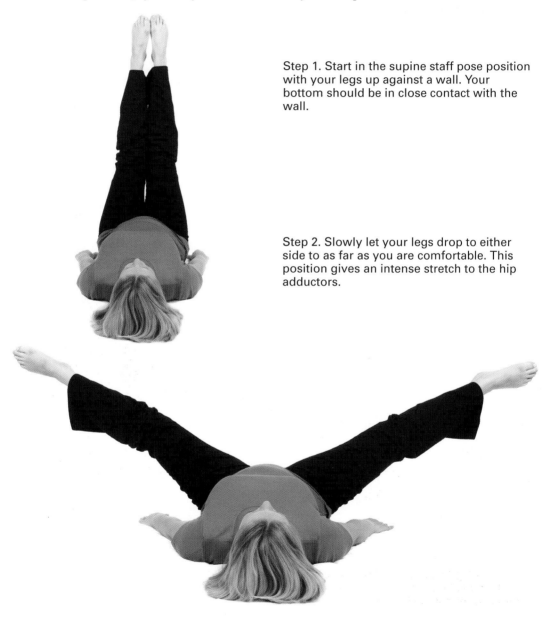

Step 1. Start in the supine staff pose position with your legs up against a wall. Your bottom should be in close contact with the wall.

Step 2. Slowly let your legs drop to either side to as far as you are comfortable. This position gives an intense stretch to the hip adductors.

Shoulder Stand and Plough Poses

These shoulder stand exercises are the most extreme inverted poses presented in this book and are not recommended for begin- ners. They carry a number of contraindica- tions (see Chapter 2). Therefore, it is recom- mended that you ensure that you are fit to participate in these exercises. If you are unsure, you should seek professional medical advice first. If you feel discomfort in

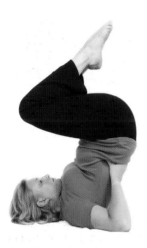

Step 1. Start by lying on your back with your knees bent. Then, keeping your legs bent, bring your legs up so that your knees are over your head. Support your lower back with your hands. Make sure that you are comfortable in this position before moving on to the next step.

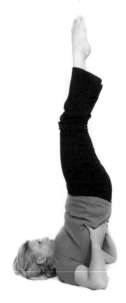

Step 2. Slowly raise your legs and straighten them. You are aiming to bring your legs in line with your shoulders. Keep your feet together.

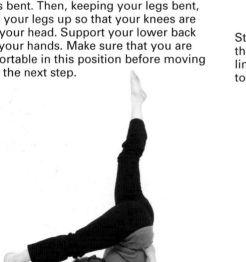

Step 3. Place one leg on the ground behind you, while keeping the other leg pointing upwards. (Repeat on the other side.)

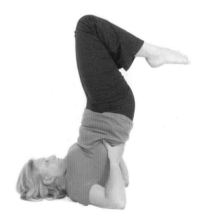

Step 4. Bring both legs together again and pointing upwards, and then bend at the knees. Keep your feet together.

any of these poses then come out of them immediately and inform your instructor.

These exercises are good for developing strength and flexibility in your neck and back, and preparing you for the more difficult head- and handstands. You should not feel any pressure in your neck. Once you are in the pose, focus on breathing slowly and deeply. Step two is the basic shoulder stand and the position shown in step six is called the plough pose.

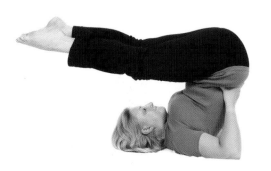

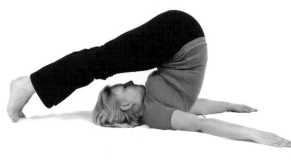

Step 5. Straighten your legs above you once more and then slowly bring them down over your head, keeping them straight. Stop when they are parallel to the ground. Keep your feet together.

Step 6. Place your feet on the ground, with your toes touching the ground. Straighten your arms and extend them on the ground with the palms down and the fingers pointing backwards. This is the plough pose.

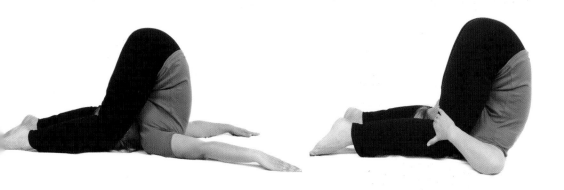

Step 7. Place your knees on the ground. The tops of your feet should be in contact with the ground also.

Step 8. Bring your knees in closer to your body; you can use your hands to help you. Focus on your breathing in this position, since it may feel quite constricted in this pose.

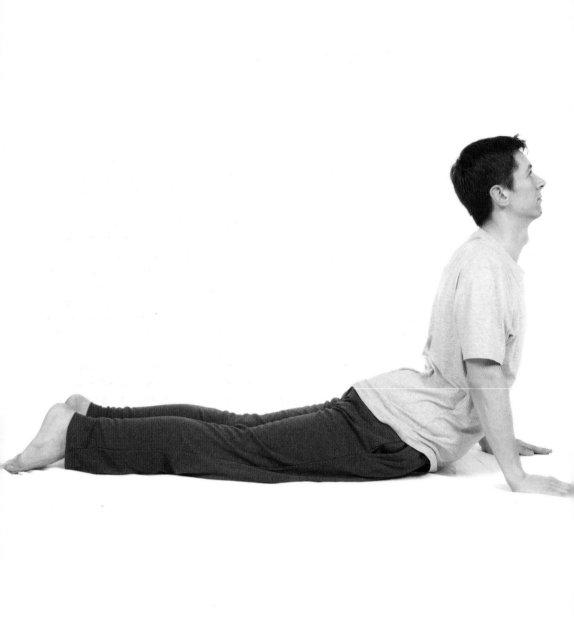

8 Floor Exercises

There are many floor exercises in yoga and they can form some of the most interesting and enjoyable shapes with your body. This chapter starts with the child pose, a simple closed pose that is both relaxing and calming. It can be used either between other more demanding yoga poses, as a way of giving the body a short break between exercises, or it can be used at the end of class for relaxation or meditation.

The dog and the cat pose are then described: these are often used as gentle exercises for relieving strain in the back. You can use these two exercises in combination by performing a PNF stretching sequence that can feel very rejuvenating. These two exercises are also useful as gentler exercises to use at the start of a session. The remaining poses described in this chapter are more challenging, most of them working the muscles in the abdomen and the back, as well as forming some unusual shapes with the body. They are a great addition to any yoga session, nearer the end of the class, forming some challenging poses to practise before relaxation. The latter poses in this chapter require much strength in order to be able to hold these poses. You can use these poses to build up your strength or to work on your flexibility depending on how you use them. The final three poses in this chapter work on your lower back flexibility and your quadriceps. There are relatively few simple exercises that can work the muscles in the front of the legs, so if this is an area that you are looking to develop, then these exercises will help you.

Child Pose

This is an excellent exercise with which to relax the body. It is good at refreshing the body after more demanding exercises, particularly exercises that arch the lower back. This pose can be used as part of the final relaxation sequence in a class or it is a good pose to use between more demanding poses as a way of having a break and clearing the mind, while resting the body.

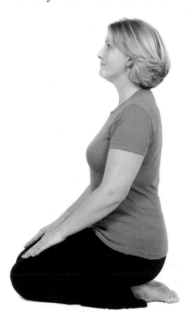

Step 1. Start in a kneeling position with your feet tucked underneath you and your back upright. Make sure that your feet are together and that your knees are together. Your gaze should be parallel to the ground.

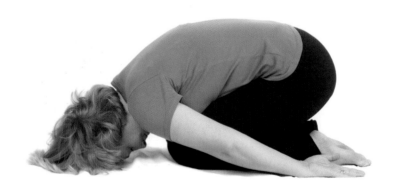

Step 2. Bend forward from your pelvic region and bring your arms to rest by your side. Rest your head down on the ground in front of you. The tops of your hands should be on the ground.

Extended Child Pose

As the name suggests, this version of the child pose adds an extension to the basic pose by stretching the arms out in front of you. This pose has the added benefit of working the shoulders and the back while in this relaxing position. This exercise can also be done with the knees wide apart, allowing the upper body to rest closer to the ground between the knees.

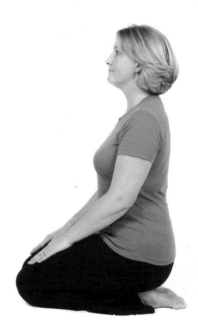

Step 1. Start in a kneeling position with your feet tucked underneath you and your back upright. Make sure that your feet are together and that your knees are together. Your gaze should be parallel to the ground.

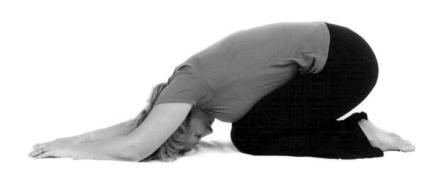

Step 2. Rest forward and bring your forearms to rest in front of you on the ground. Rest your head down on the ground in front of you. Your fingers should point forwards.

123

Dog Pose

This is a gentle back exercise and a good place to start any exercises that work the back more intensely. This pose can be combined into a PNF sequence with the cat pose working the back alternately in both directions. The key is to make the movements to get into the pose gentle and slow and then holding the position once in place. This exercise will actively work its way along the whole of the spine.

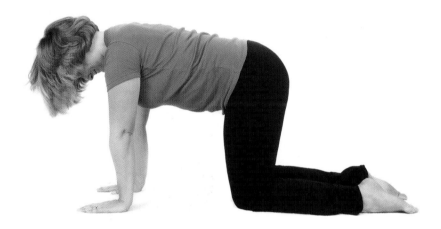

Step 1. Start in a position from all fours on the ground. Ensure that your knees and palms are a hip-width apart and keep your back straight. Your fingers should point forwards.

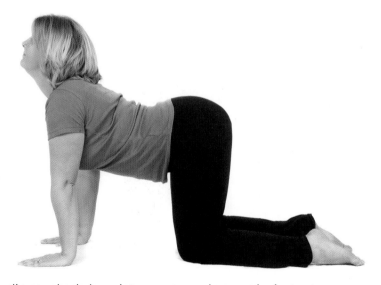

Step 2. Gently dip your back down into a concave shape and raise your head, lifting your gaze. Keep your arms straight.

Cat Pose

This pose is similar to the dog pose, except that it works the back in the opposite direction. This makes it a good exercise to combine with the dog pose to form a PNF sequence. The key is to make the movements to get into the pose gentle and slow and then holding the position once in place. This exercise will actively work its way along the whole of the spine.

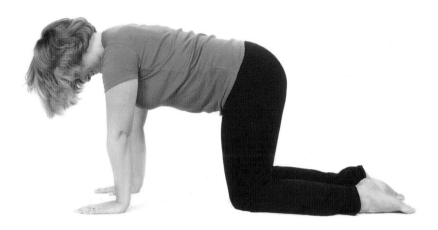

Step 1. Start in a position from all fours on the ground. Ensure that your knees and palms are a hip-width apart and keep your back straight. Your fingers should point forwards.

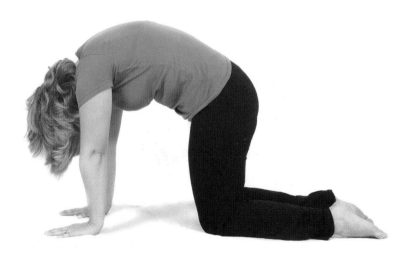

Step 2. Gently lift your back up into a convex shape and drop your head down. Keep your arms straight.

Locust Pose

This pose may look simple and yet it requires good strength in order to hold this position for any length of time. It is an excellent exercise for working both the abdomen and the lower back muscles. Due to the difficulty of the pose, and because it can be quite tiring, it is worth trying this pose for, say, five counts and then resting back down to step one before attempting the pose again. Practising this around three times in a row is recommended.

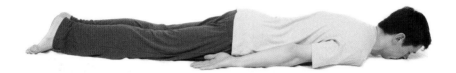

Step 1. Lie on your front with your feet together and your arms resting by your side. The tops of your hands should be in contact with the ground.

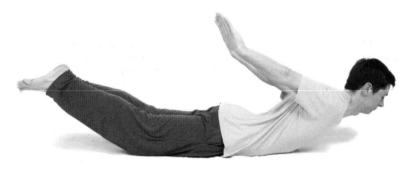

Step 2. Slowly lift your legs and your upper body off the ground as high as you are able. Let your arms rise up behind you. Focus on using your core muscles to help you to hold this position.

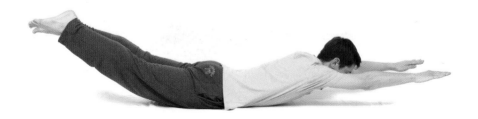

Variant: Raise your arms up in front of you with your fingers pointing forwards and your palms down.

Cobra Pose

The cobra pose is also known as the serpent pose. Like the locust pose, this exercise works the back. In addition, however, it requires arm strength in order to hold the position. Performing this pose gives a wonderful sense of opening and it is a delight to perform on sunny days as it has a sense of basking in the sun about it. This exercise is an excellent one for working the spine. Also, due to the weight being supported on the hands, it can help to strengthen the arms.

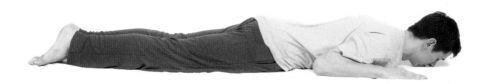

Step 1. Lie on your front with your feet a hip-width apart and your palms resting on the ground next to your shoulders. Let your feet point behind you, so that the tops of your feet touch the ground. Your fingers should point forwards.

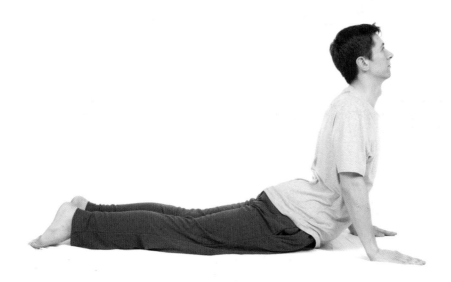

Step 2. Slowly lift your upper body off the ground, keeping your hips as close to the ground as possible. Keep your neck in line with your back and lift your gaze upwards.

Plank Pose

This pose is another one that demands upper body strength. It is particularly recommended if you are looking to strengthen your arms. Again, this pose is more difficult than it looks. Due to its difficulty and because it can be quite tiring, it is worth trying this pose for, say, five counts and then resting back down to step one before attempting the pose again. Practising this around three times in a row is recommended.

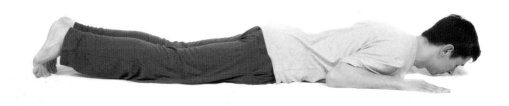

Step 1. Lie on your front with your feet a hip-width apart and your palms resting on the ground next to your shoulders. Keep your toes on the ground. Your fingers should point forwards.

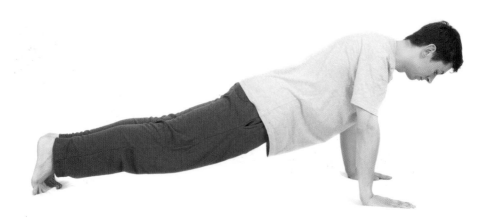

Step 2. Lift your body off the ground while keeping your whole body straight. Keep your head in line with your back and keep your gaze down.

Sage Pose

This exercise builds on the plank pose and is more difficult, as the weight is transferred from both hands onto one. These steps not only require upper body strength, they also require good balance. These exercises are very demanding, and so again it is worth trying this pose for, say, five counts and then resting back down to step one before attempting the pose again. Practising this around three times in a row is recommended. Remember to repeat on both sides.

This pose strengthens the wrists and the arms. Try to keep your balance while letting the muscles in the arms do the majority of the work. It is better for beginners to work on getting comfortable with step three before moving onto the complete pose.

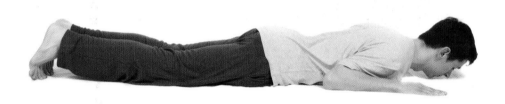

Step 1. Lie on your front with your feet a hip-width apart and your palms resting on the ground next to your shoulders. Keep your toes on the ground. Your fingers should point forwards.

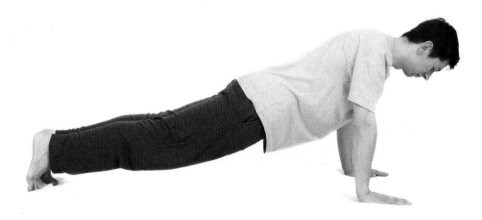

Step 2. Lift your body off the ground while keeping your whole body straight. Keep your head in line with your back and keep your gaze down.

129

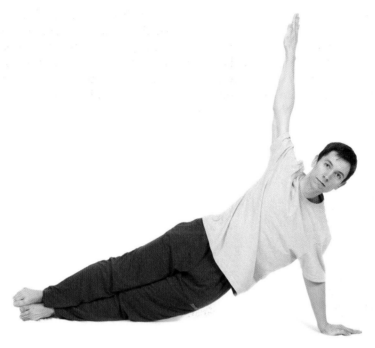

Step 3. Rotate your body to the side, rest one foot on top of the other and raise your non-supporting arm so that it points vertically upwards.

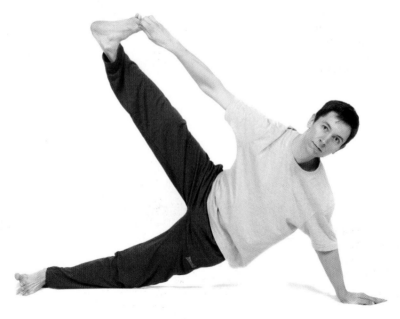

Step 4. Slowly lift your non-supporting leg up as high as you can while keeping it straight. Hold your foot with your hand.

Bow Pose

In this pose, the body forms the shape of a bow. This exercise is quite challenging, requiring strength in the abdomen. It is also a good exercise for improving flexibility in the spine. Again, this pose is more difficult than it looks. Due to the difficulty of the pose, and because it can be quite tiring, it is worth trying this pose for, say, five counts and then resting back down to step one before attempting the pose again. Practising this around three times in a row is recommended.

Step 1. Lie on your front with your feet a hip-width apart and your hands resting on the ground next to your hips. Let your feet point behind you so that the tops of your feet touch the ground. The back of your hands should be in contact with the ground.

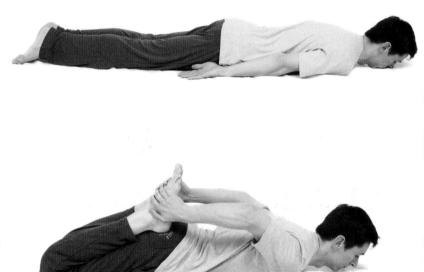

Step 2. Hold your feet with your hands, while resting your feet on your bottom. Keep your feet a hip-width apart.

Step 3. Keeping hold of your feet, lift your legs and as much of your upper body off the ground as possible. Focus on using your core muscles to help you to hold this position.

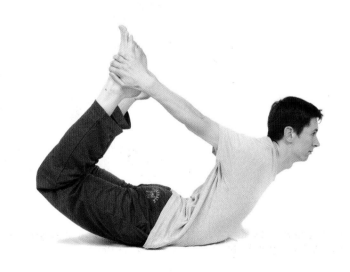

Wheel Pose

This pose requires much spine flexibility and upper body strength in order to hold the position. Again, this pose is more difficult than it looks. Due to the difficulty of the pose and that it can be quite tiring, it is worth trying this pose for, say, five counts and then resting back down to step one before attempting the pose again. Practising this around three times in a row is recommended.

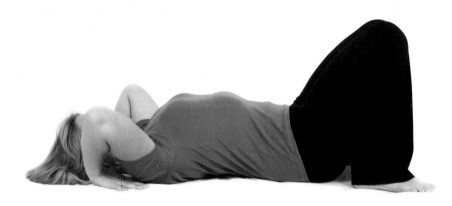

Step 1. Lie on your back and bring your feet and hands in towards your torso, placing your palms and feet flat on the ground. Your feet should be a hip-width apart and your fingers should point backwards.

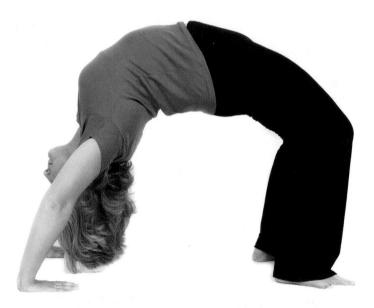

Step 2. Slowly lift your body off the ground, aiming for the body to form a smooth curve.

Camel Pose

The camel pose is good for working the quadriceps. There are many exercises that work the hamstrings but far fewer that work these muscles. This muscle group is often quite tight as it is not normally used in everyday activities or sports. Therefore you may find stretching this muscle quite difficult. For this reason, it is best to perform these steps with great care in order to minimize the risk of injury.

The quadriceps are essential muscles to work on if you aspire to be able to do the front splits. This sequence is a gentle way of stretching the quadriceps and is suitable for beginners. It is best to work through the sequence and stop at whichever step you feel you have reached your maximum. Since this muscle group is normally very tight, do not push yourself too hard and overstretch.

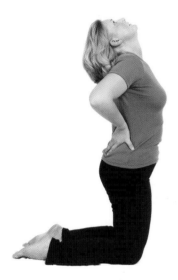

Step 1. With your knees on the ground, stay upright, with your hips in line with your knees. Then support your lower back and look upwards. Your feet and knees should be a hip-width apart.

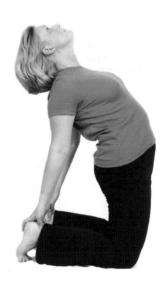

Step 2. Raise your feet onto your toes and rest your hands on your heels. Keep your arms straight.

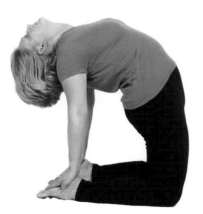

Step 3. Place the tops of your feet back onto the ground and place your hands onto the soles of your feet, with the fingers pointing in the same direction as your toes.

Pigeon Pose

This pose works the lower back and the quadriceps. Use the step by step approach to help guide you to how far you can proceed with this exercise. The final step opens up the chest and should feel refreshing once this pose has been mastered.

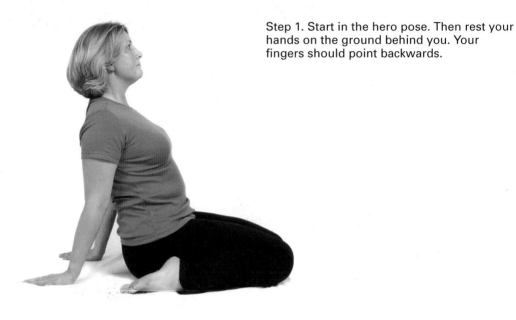

Step 1. Start in the hero pose. Then rest your hands on the ground behind you. Your fingers should point backwards.

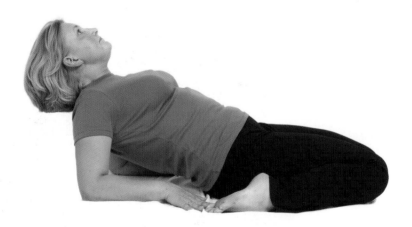

Step 2. Place your forearms down on the ground behind you, with your palms in contact with the ground. Do not let your knees lift off the ground.

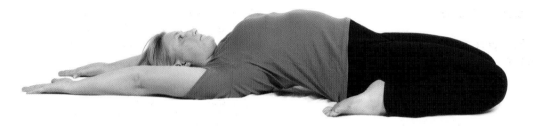

Step 3. Place your arms down on the ground behind you and extend them. The back of your hands should be on the ground and your fingers should point backwards. Do not let your knees lift off the ground.

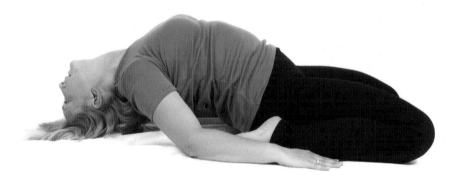

Step 4. Place the top of your head down on the ground behind you. Bring your forearms back onto the ground to support you.

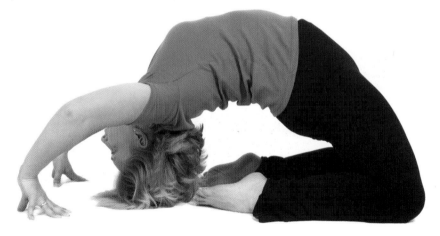

Step 5. Work towards resting your head onto the soles of your feet. Use your hands to help you to bring your head in closer.

Quadriceps Stretch

This quadriceps stretch is very effective in isolating that muscle group, enabling you to focus on this area. Since so few exercises are good at working this muscle group, this makes this stretch a very important exercise to incorporate into your practice. It is more difficult to achieve than the camel and pigeon poses, which also work the quadriceps.

You can control the stretch by levering the leg in as far as is comfortable. This exercise will help you to carefully monitor your progress with this muscle group. It works towards the royal pigeon pose, where the head is moved backwards to rest onto the sole of the foot. Remember to repeat this exercise on both sides of the body.

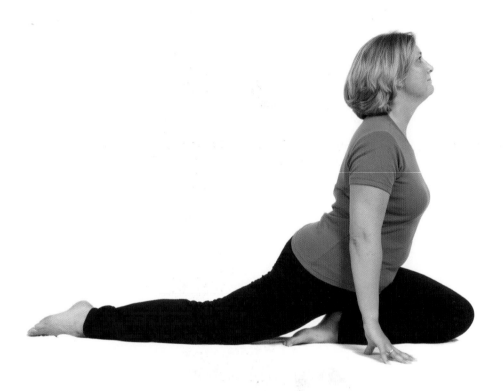

Step 1. Start in a kneeling position. Then push one leg back behind you, while keeping as low as possible. Ensure that your back is as upright as possible. Pull your shoulders slightly back to help open up the chest.

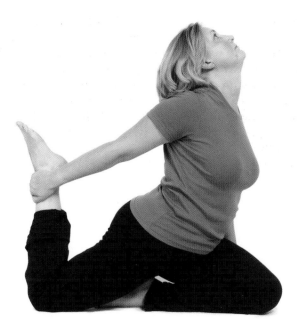

Step 2. Bring the rear leg in towards your body by bending at the knee and reach around with your hand to hold your foot.

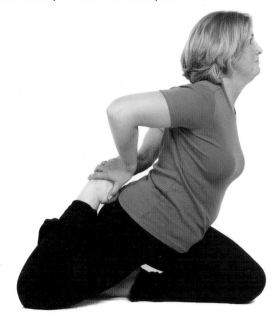

Step 3. Hold your foot with both hands and bring your foot in towards your body and rest it on your bottom. Try not to lean the upper body forward in this position.

Sun Salutation

No yoga book would be complete without a sun salutation sequence. This exercise works through a range of poses in a circular sequence. On its own, it forms a mini workout and is often used by instructors to get students warmed up for the class. It contains a good range of exercises that work most of the major muscles groups in the body. In fact, only the hip adductors do not get much of a workout from this routine. For this reason, the sun salutation is a good workout for the posterior and the anterior of the body.

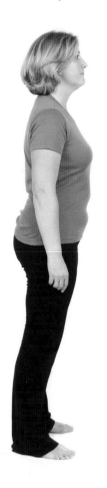

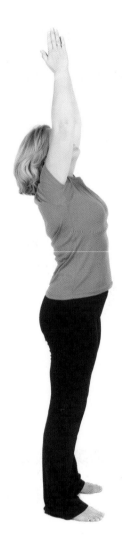

Step 1. Start in the basic standing position.

Step 2. Reach up, bringing your palms together and keeping your arms straight.

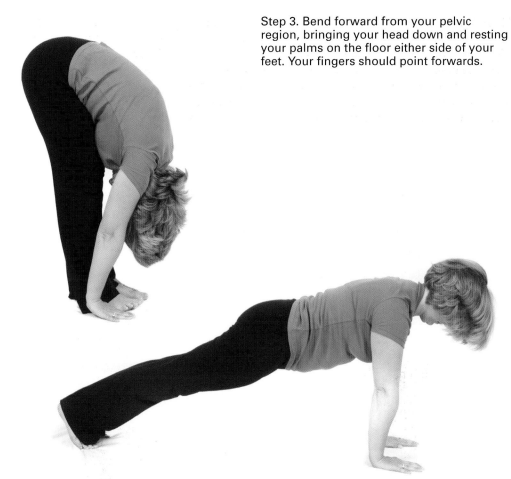

Step 3. Bend forward from your pelvic region, bringing your head down and resting your palms on the floor either side of your feet. Your fingers should point forwards.

Step 4. Jump back, into the plank pose.

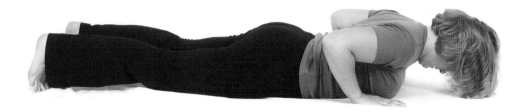

Step 5. Bend at the elbows and bring your upper body down. Your fingers should point forwards. This position is known as the four limbed staff pose.

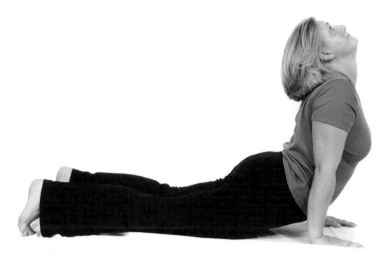

Step 6. Push up into an upward-facing dog pose. Keep your hips pushed down. Lift your gaze upwards.

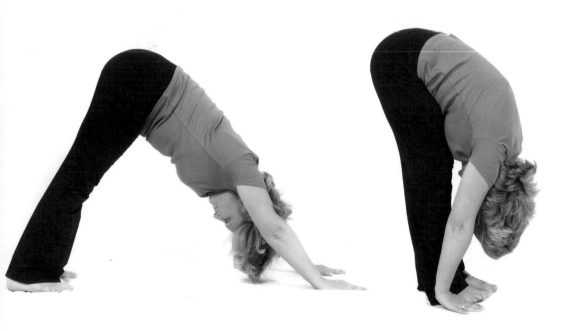

Step 7. Push with your arms to move yourself into a downward-facing dog pose.

Step 8. Bend forward from your pelvic region, bringing your head down and resting your palms on the floor either side of your feet. Your fingers should point forwards.

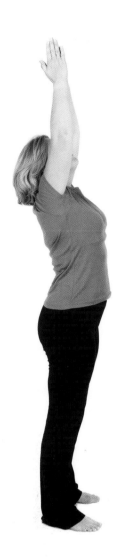

Step 9. Reach up, bringing your palms together and keeping your arms straight.

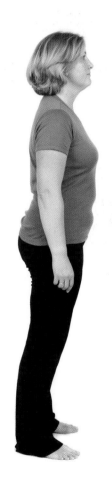

Step 10. Finish in the basic standing position.

141

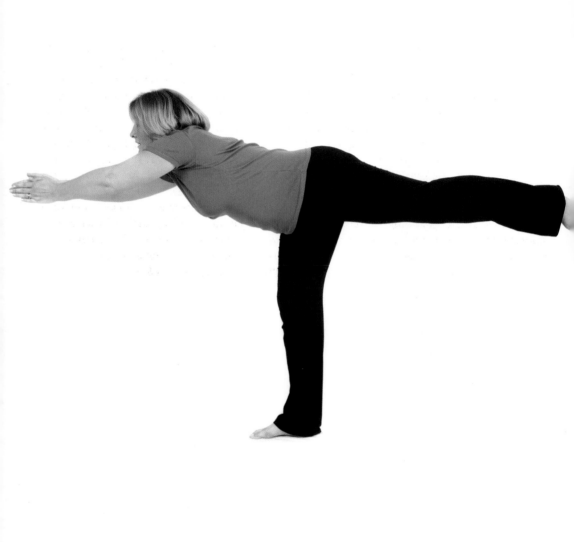

9 Session Planning

The step by step approach presented in Chapters 4 to 8 is designed to help you identify your individual development needs. Even without such an analysis, students often ask what exercises they can do to help them focus on a particular part of their body, be that the back, the legs or some other part. In this chapter, you will be able to use that information to help select exercises and plan sessions that will match your needs.

To help you to plan, a yoga session is described as being composed of four stages: preparation, fundamentals, challenge and relaxation. Within each stage, there are a number of suggested sample exercise sequences that you could use to compose your session. One way of staying excited about your training and making it fun is to ensure that each lesson contains some variety and something fresh. Sessions should be enjoyable, and so varying the difficulty level, so that there are some sections that are relaxing, some fun and others that are challenging, will give you a good balanced lesson. Therefore you should use the session planning tool to mix and match sequences and exercises.

The suggested sequences are shown in an easy to follow format, enabling quick reference during training. (For full details of the exercises and variations to make the poses simpler or more difficult, see Chapters 4 to 8.)

Planning a Session

Once you have identified the areas that you wish to develop, either through your own experience or by using the step by step approach in the preceding chapters, you can use the session planning table as a guide to how to structure a session. You should plan on the session lasting between one and two hours, depending, of course, on how much time you spend within each stage and each pose. The session planner and stages shown should help you to get started in putting together a suitable lesson.

The session is divided into four stages. In the preparation stage, you are looking to perform some simple exercises that will help to bring your focus on to your training and to slow down and deepen your breathing. These exercises will also help by starting to get your body ready for more intense poses. The fundamentals stage is designed for you to work through a core set of exercises that will engage many of your major muscle groups. They should help by limbering you up, ready for the more challenging poses. The challenge stage is, as the name suggests, composed of exercises that should challenge your ability level and help to push forward your training. It is not essential to be able to complete the full pose in these sequences. They are merely intended to push you a little further, adding some variety and fun to your lesson. It is recommended that you end the session with a stage of relaxation. You can either choose simple poses to hold and allow you to focus on your breathing or you can choose slightly more difficult poses to hold, which you have already mastered and find effortlessly comfortable. Many of the exercises where you lie on your back can be suitable for this stage.

Using the Session Planner

In the session planner table, there are a number of recommended sequences under each stage. This is so that you can pick and mix sequences as appropriate to you. You can pick any number of sequences from each stage. It just depends on how long you intend your session to last and how quickly you perform each exercise. Each sequence contains a number of recommended poses that work on a particular area. You can either practise the poses shown or use either easier or more difficult variations (see Chapters 4 to 8). When using the session planner, bear in mind the following:

- It is recommended that a lesson should last between one and two hours. You can choose how long to spend on each stage, depending on what you are trying to achieve.
- You do not have to incorporate each stage into your session plan each time.
- Equally, you do not have to incorporate each pose, in a given sequence, into your session. They are merely recommendations.
- Try to have a good mix of sequences so that your session is both challenging and fun.
- Remember to punctuate your session with the simple exercises, such as shaking off and flexing the knees (see Chapter 4), as appropriate.

Session Planner

Stage 1: Preparation	Stage 2: Fundamentals	Stage 3: Challenge	Stage 4: Relaxation
Neck	Posterior – Simple	Core – Simple	Simple
Wrists	Hip adductors – Simple	Core – Advanced	Intermediate
Ankles and knees	Triangle routine	Back – Advanced	Advanced
Arms	Warrior routine	Back – Rotation	With movement
Back – Simple	Sun salutation	Posterior – Advanced	
Legs – Simple		Quadriceps	
		Hip adductors – Advanced	
		Balancing	
		Arms	
		Shoulder stand routine	

Once you have selected the sequences that you wish to incorporate into your session, you can then use the following sequences for the details on which poses are recommended. These spreads should act as quick reference guides for your use during training. (For full details of the exercises and variations to make the poses simpler or more difficult, see Chapters 4 to 8.)

PREPARATION SEQUENCES

Neck

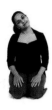

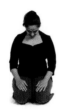

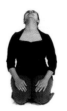

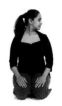

| Head to the side | Head forward | Head back | Head rotation |

Wrists

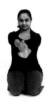

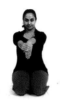

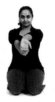

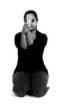

| Wrist flexor | Wrist extensor | Wrist and forearm extensor | Wrist rotation |

Ankles and knees

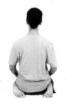

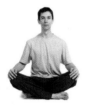

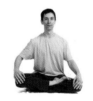

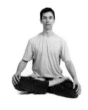

| Hero pose | Easy pose | Half lotus pose | Lotus pose |

Arms

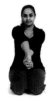

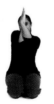

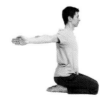

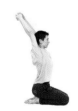

| Forearm rotation | Forearms entwined | Arm rotation | Arm lift – front |

Arms *(continued)*

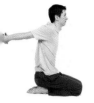 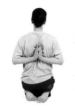 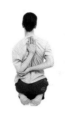 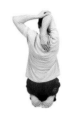 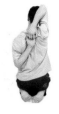

| Arm lift – behind | Palms together | Elbow up | Elbow down | Hands together |

Back – simple

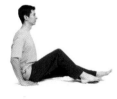 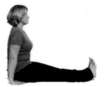 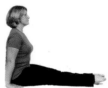 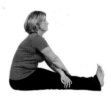

| Side stretch | Dog pose | Cat pose | Cobra pose | Extended child pose |

Legs – Simple

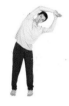 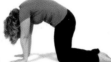 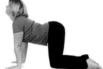 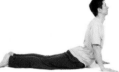 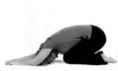

| Flex the knees | Pull the feet back | Point the feet | Simple posterior pose |

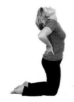 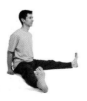

Simple camel pose   Angle pose

FUNDAMENTALS SEQUENCES

Posterior – Simple

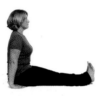 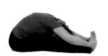 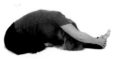

Simple single leg
Pull the feet back Posterior pose Head to knee pose Standing forward bend forward bend

Hip adductors – Simple

 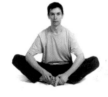 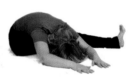 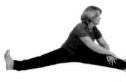

Angle pose   Simple sitting stretch   Head to knee pose I   Seated angle pose

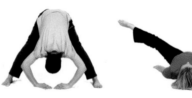

Feet apart forward bend   Supine angle pose

Triangle routine

Warrior routine

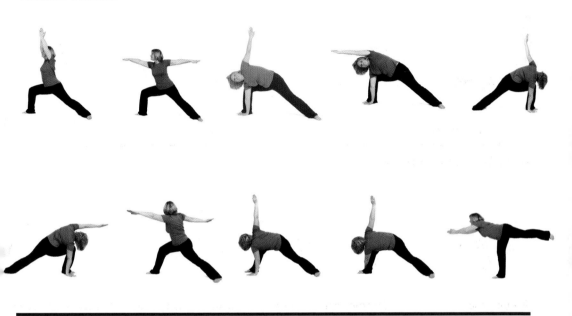

Sun salutation

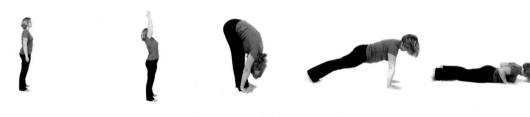

Starting position   Reach up   Forward bend   Plank pose   Four limbed staff pose

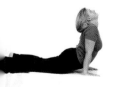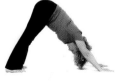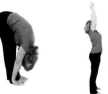

pward-facing dog   Downward-facing dog   Forward bend   Reach up   Starting position

CHALLENGE SEQUENCES I

Core – Simple

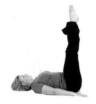
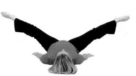
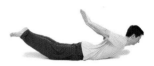

Supine staff pose   Supine angle pose   Locust pose

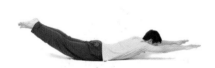
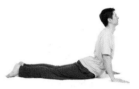

Locust pose variation   Cobra pose

Core – Advanced

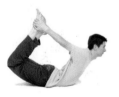
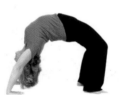
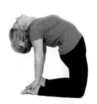
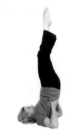

Bow pose   Wheel pose   Camel pose   Shoulder stand

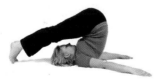
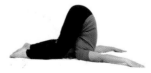

Plough pose   Plough pose variation

Back – Advanced

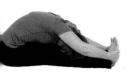

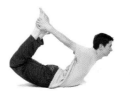

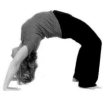

Posterior pose   Forward bend   Bow pose   Wheel pose

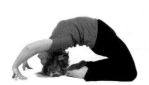

Camel pose   Pigeon pose variation

Back rotation

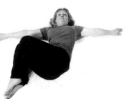

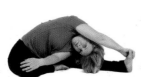

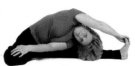

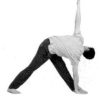

Knees to chest   Revolved head to knee pose   Seated gate pose   Rotated triangle pose

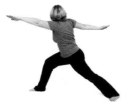

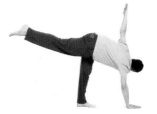

Rotated warrior II pose   Rotated half moon pose

CHALLENGE SEQUENCES II

Posterior – Advanced

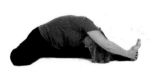 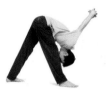 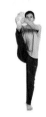

Head to knee II pose Simple single leg forward bend Extended hand to toe pose

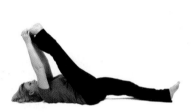 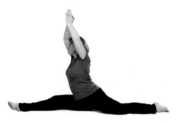

Supine hand to toe pose   Hanuman pose

Quadriceps

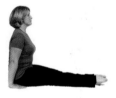 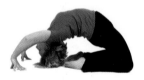

Point the feet   Quadriceps stretch   Pigeon pose

 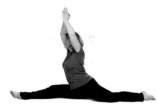 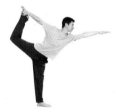

Camel pose   Hanuman pose   Standing half bow pose

Hip adductors – Advanced

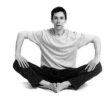
Sitting stretch

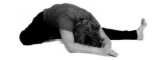
Head to knee II pose variant

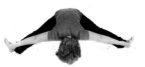
Seated angle pose

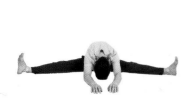
Feet apart forward bend

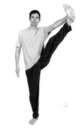
Side extended hand to toe pose

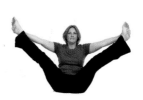
Lifted angle pose

Balancing

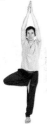

Tree pose

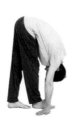
Simple single leg forward bend pose

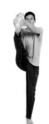
Extended hand to toe pose

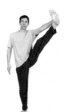
Side extended hand to toe pose

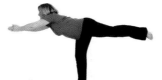
Warrior III pose

Half moon pose

153

CHALLENGE SEQUENCES III

Balancing *(continued)*

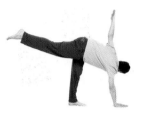

Rotated half moon pose

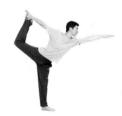

Standing half bow pose

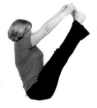

Double toe hold pose

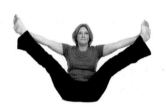

Lifted angle pose

Arms

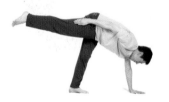

Half moon pose

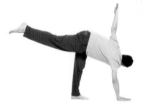

Rotated half moon pose

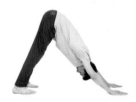

Downward-facing dog pose

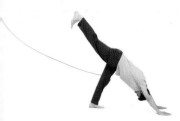

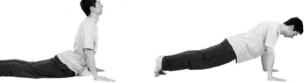

One-legged downward-facing dog pose   Cobra pose   Plank pose

Arms *(continued)*

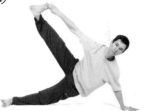

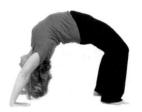

Sage pose   Wheel pose

Shoulder stand routine

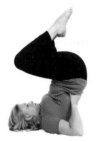 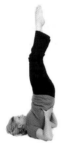 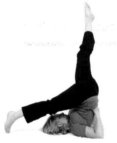 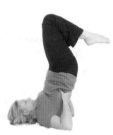

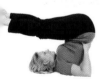 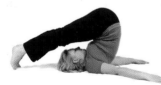 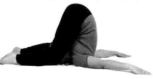 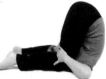

155

RELAXATION SEQUENCES

Simple

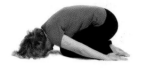

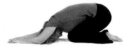

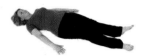

| Child pose | Extended child pose | Corpse pose |

Intermediate

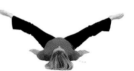

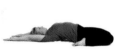

Easy pose   Hero pose   Supine angle pose   Simple pigeon pos

Advanced

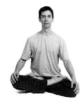 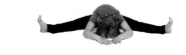 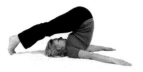

Lotus pose   Seated angle pose   Plough pose

With movement

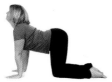 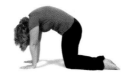 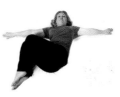

Dog pose   Cat pose   Knees to chest

Bibliography

Brown, C., *The Yoga Bible: The Definitive Guide to Yoga Postures* (Godsfield Press, 2003)

Iyengar, B.K.S., *Light on Yoga* (Thorsons, 1991), *Light on the Yoga Sutras of Patanjali* (Thorsons, 2002)

Lamb, D.R., *Physiology of Exercise: Responses and Adoptions* (Macmillan Publishing Company, 1984)

Norris, C.M., *The Complete Guide to Stretching* (A & C Black Publishers Limited, 2001)

Worthington, V., *A History of Yoga* (Routledge, 1982)

Index